hy·po·der·mal

Beating Suicide and Depression

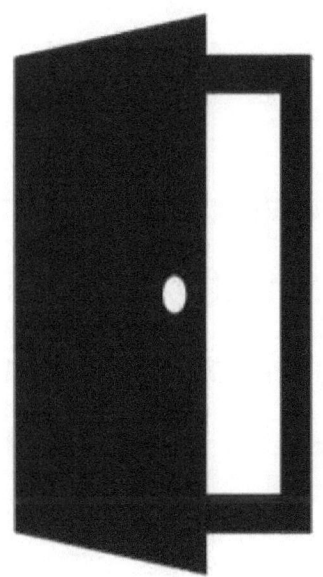

By

Dark Myer

hy·po·der·mal

For Brownie the Wonder Dog
It has been fifty years, old friend
I still miss you every single day

hy·po·der·mal

con·tents

pref·ace 1

o·ver·view 5

trig·gers 8

in·flu·ence 24

com·mit·ment 35

grasp·ing 43

di·chot·o·my 50

re·spite 57

os·cil·la·tion 69

sab·o·tage 83

e·piph·a·ny 104

fail·ure.. 118

suc·cess 129

hy·po·der·mal

hope·ful 133

five·true·things 137

short·cut 140

dis·til·la·tion 142

hy·po·der·mal

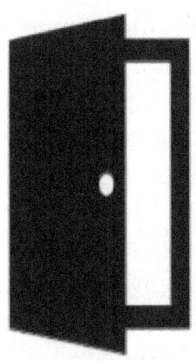

pref·ace

Why would you chop off your own arm? It is stupid, it hurts, and it's permanently debilitating. It is a very easy task to avoid chopping off your arm. You do it all day long, every day. In fact, it is very easy to stop thinking about it. Try it yourself. It is a simple effort to think of anything but chopping off your arm. Think of a cactus or a mountain. See, it was that easy. And you are not even tempted to spend a few seconds actually considering the removal of your arm. You simply move on without any mental or emotional struggle at all.

The reason it is easy to avoid thinking one second, much less actually considering such a crazy thought is because you know for an absolute certainty it is stupid. There is no question in your mind like, "Hmmm, should I chop this off or not?" You know there is no upside and it is crystal clear you will not be better off by doing so. You unquestioningly know this profound truth regarding chopping or not chopping off your perfectly healthy, useful arm and you won't actually consider it. It is a waste of time.

There are lots of truths you know at least that well or even better. Lots. But what are we missing? What profound truth have we yet to find? What wonder lies hidden among

hy·po·der·mal

the lies? Trouble most often comes our way when we are missing key information or experiences regarding a profound truth. I was missing some profound truths for most of my lifetime and had no clue that was the case. This is the story of uncovering profound truths so that you won't cut off your arm, so to speak.

Sitting in a dark room with a loaded pistol, I knew suicide and its ugly cousin, depression, really were matters of life and death. Cliché, but true. I know because I have danced with these devils and spent the majority of my sixty-year life (assuming I do not exceed 119) failing at everything worth doing. Sure, I enjoyed temporary successes, but they were all obliterated by mistakes and malfunctions until each and every lifeless carcass flopped down into my favorite darkness.

Like many suffering with depression, I presented a consistently upbeat face and a practiced smile to all who knew me while just below the skin, I was decaying and rotting. Fortunately, hope is a stubborn, death-resistant creature and at least in my case, it tenaciously fought for my survival, refusing to be snuffed out in spite of all I could do.

Along my two-faced path, there have been hundreds of well-meaning people clamoring after me, convinced of my success, something I knew to be utterly false. Those poor fools. Their attempts were valiant, but each and every inane word smashed against my certainty stone. The concrete conviction of my total and perfect failure was so total and perfect that I could not have been shaken without something outside my thought prison.

Fortunately, this very thing happened just as both hope and I were pulling the plug. I never saw it coming, but in the blink of an eye my runaway tragedy derailed, demolished my certainty, and left me breathlessly willing to live. This is my own story of life and death, my internal workings, the guts so to speak of my thoughts, emotions, and feelings riding a

hy·po·der·mal

sixty-year failure train with regular stops at Depression Depot and Suicide Junction.

Although this is my story, it is not written for me. I already know how it ends and the butler didn't do it. This story is for you. A kind of how-to approach to unloading some lethal anchors hanging around your neck. This book is in no way intended to be autobiographical, although that is exactly the delivery method. Using my own falls and recoveries to present a do-it-yourself approach that has absolutely worked for at least one person, I am saying if I can do it, you can too.

My words walk a razor's edge between a narcissistic, self-serving tirade and a pity-seeking brag-fest of my scars and bruises. There is a sweet spot right between those two extremes and that is where I am aiming. If I do my job right, you will not think me crazy when I declare at the end of our journey, "Constant failure is my greatest success" and you might even join me. Don't worry, skepticism is an important part of the journey.

You are right, "constant failure is my greatest success" sounds completely counter-intuitive to our modern and super-smart soothsayers, but I assure you, I am not handing out repair patches that fall off after a while or a flavor-of-the-month fix that disappears with your hopes. There are some truths that are so profound that once you know them, really know them, you can't backslide. Here is one just to get you started: "Success has nothing to do with outcomes and if you think it does, you couldn't be more wrong." Doesn't look like much of a profound, life-altering truth, does it? Believe it or not, this little ditty can not only save your life for the rest of your life, it provides a peace that you will never, ever lose. Ever.

Truth is all around us, but profound truths have the ability to permanently fill you with hope even as your life remains full of misery. I know it is possible for such truths to affect irreversible changes and save a life in the process.

hy·po·der·mal

I am living proof and I assure you, this is very doable stuff. No special skills or beliefs are required. Just a willing heart. But, it has to be a truly willing heart. We have to leave the area of fake or shallow efforts behind. Wishing is not sufficient.

This is a brutally true and personal story, although I have omitted the names of both the guilty and the innocent. If any part of these words release you from your successes and helps you embrace your failures, please feel free to make that part your own. Yeah, it sounds crazy, but stay with me and you'll see it is not. Most importantly, if this makes any sense to you, once a profound truth gets a hold of you, you will no longer ever be afraid to live inside your own skin, or in other words, hypodermal.

Dark Myer, Complete Failure

hy·po·der·mal

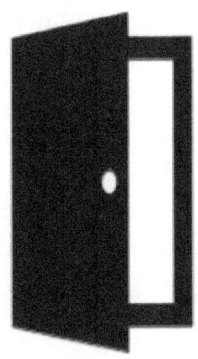

o·ver·view

I am only an expert in suicide and depression as a participant. I have no credentials and no train of academic letters trailing after my name. In spite of this, I think I can speak with some understanding and authority from an insider's perspective, so here goes.

As far as I can tell, there are three kinds of suicides and two kinds of depressions, each one based on different driving compulsions or some combination thereof. Understanding each compulsion is essential to uncovering the root causes of these menaces, otherwise we are just slapping patches on symptoms and not curing diseases. The three suicides and two depressions are:

1. Mental Health Driven Suicide
2. Attention Driven Suicide
3. Lie Driven Suicide
1. Chemical Depression
2. Circumstantial Depression

Of course, it is possible to have more than one of these with some unfortunate souls possessing all five. They each have unique characteristics and it is my opinion they need to be recognized individually in order to understand and effectively deal with them. What follows are some short observations of each and the role this book plays regarding them:

Mental Health Driven Suicides are way out of the purview of this book. This is an arena belonging to experts and people a whole lot smarter than me. The preventative treatments seem to be largely confined to drugs and/or some system of restraint.

Attention Driven Suicides can have some of the same root causes as Lie-Driven Suicides (which will be addressed in the coming chapters) and often appear to cluster around a single misconception: The belief that outcomes can be controlled when in fact, they are not controllable at all. Sure, we can influence an outcome with our inputs, but that still doesn't give us control over the result. In believing otherwise, we are often infected with hopelessness, usually driven by a faulty definition of failure or success. Taking responsibility for an outcome in the form of guilt or credit is tricky business and in particular, seems to afflict our youth or less experienced adults. This book will touch on some key points, but I suspect preventing this type of suicide requires additional expertise or at least a more focused approach.

Lie Driven Suicide and Circumstantial Depression are the targets of this book. As you will see, both of these deceivers can be defeated once we identify exactly what we are fighting. Warning: There are no shortcuts, but that doesn't mean good things can't happen very, very quickly. Don't be surprised when they do.

Chemical Depression is also out of the purview of this book. It is real, but there are some associated aspects of concern. Balancing chemicals among so many different sets of circumstances has got to be a hit or miss process a great deal of the time. There are simply too many independent variables. Additionally, I personally have been misdiagnosed or more likely, some key contributors were

hy·po·der·mal

missed in my diagnosis. The only thing I can say regarding this disease is to urge consideration that a lot of depression is at least partly circumstantially driven and the root causes can be, and often are, ancient and deeply hidden – **sometimes masked by the drugs themselves**. Until root causes are exposed and addressed, at least in the case of Circumstantial Depression, only symptoms are being treated and the underlying drivers very likely remain secret. No one can permanently solve a problem by only dealing with symptoms, unless they are an extremely lucky guesser. I don't believe in luck or guessing when it comes to these deadly diseases.

Now we are ready to go. Sit back, and enjoy…no, you I am not certain you will actually enjoy the ride, but I promise you, the destination is worth the few hours it takes. And who doesn't love a good underdog, come from behind story?

hy·po·der·mal

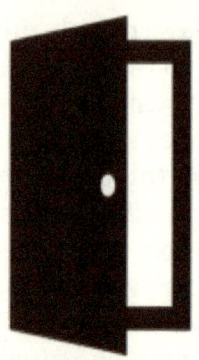

trig·gers

    I can't believe I am going to plagiarize old Chuck Dickens, but, "It was the best of times, it was the worst of times," are the most accurate words I can imagine to launch this morality tale. Coincidentally, the very best and very worst events that ever occurred in my life happened just a few days apart. I was four years old and completely unaware when the best thing transpired, oblivious to the ripples that would bounce and rebound, weaving patterns throughout my years. On the other hand, the worst thing soaked deep into me like bone cancer and I am still excavating hidden damage and rot to this very day.
    The best thing in my life didn't even happen directly to me. For most of my youth, I thought of it as anything but a best thing, it was more of a bitter imposition than anything else. My best thing happened when my agnostic father accepted religion for the first time in his adult life and I was brought along kicking and screaming into that world with him.
    Organized religion, as far as I was concerned, was something that got in the way of freedom and Sunday morning cartoons and felt more like a punishment thing more than a best thing. I am genetically inclined to vagrancy

hy·po·der·mal

and in spite of my natural opposition to all things structured, I eventually learned there was something of great worth to me in religion, but almost certainly not what you're expecting. I'll briefly touch on this topic down the road, in the meantime this chapter is devoted to misery. Oh goody.

In 1962, my mother chose to have an affair with the owner of a restaurant in which she was waitressing located in southwest Colorado. My father had been married previously and although I don't know what caused his first divorce, there were hints that his first wife had behaved similarly.

Dad did not react well to Mom's revelation. Guns were loaded, lives were threatened, and there was at least one violent altercation. Even though I witnessed much of what happened, I was only four and there was no way I could process the scenes before me.

I have a single recollection of what I believe to be the opening salvo in which my father was sitting in a chair, quietly weeping while my mother was standing stoically in front of him. My older brother was also in the room, silently cowering to one side. I was terrified. Someone was holding a baseball bat, but I have forgotten who. I am told many terrible things happened, but apparently I have misplaced or blocked my other memories.

This snapshot from my life stands as the moment, the single worst moment of my life, and the odd thing is I wasn't even a slight consideration at the time. Nobody in that room understood the deep gouges being carved inside me because everybody was fully occupied with their own pain. Dad was thirty-eight and had just lost his second wife to another man. My mother was twenty-nine and had just chosen to annihilate her first marriage, her own family, and the marriage and family of the man with whom she was having the affair. My brother was twelve years old and only he knows what kind of damage he was absorbing.

hy·po·der·mal

Somewhere later in life, I stumbled onto the fact that uncovering the root of a problem is a good thing if you want to fix or improve something. I guess I had wasted a lot of time whacking like crazy at symptoms, the leaves and branches of a problem, and it wasn't until I started addressing roots that I was finally able to make some lasting changes. It turns out that my worst moment, a large and entrenched root, will generate all sorts of unpleasant and unexpected repercussions through the ensuing decades.

There was actually a two-part schism as this root took hold. In the first, Dad, Brownie the Wonder Dog, and I left for a month long trek through Texas, Alabama, Georgia, and Florida leaving my brother and my mother to fend for themselves. When we returned to Colorado, there was another explosion between my parents after which my mother sank into some type of catatonic state, shutting off all communication and cognitive functions. I am told she never spoke or reacted to anything for some weeks or possibly even months.

Shortly before succumbing to her toxic haze, she told my father that she didn't want to keep either of her sons and that is how the two of us ended up with Dad while my mother stayed with her younger sister somewhere in the Midwest. This was schism part-two and it is my final four-year-old memory of my mother. This one is burned into my mind, starkly vivid and clear even fifty years later.

I was reaching for Mom, screaming and clawing at the back window of our car. My brother was grappling with me as I wailed and watched her fade into the distance. The last thing I saw as the dust billowed up behind our car, was Mom standing expressionless on a weather-worn porch with her arms hanging limply at her sides. Obviously, this was another terrible most worst moment, but as horrible as it was, there is another even greater worst yet to come.

You might wonder how a little boy can have more than one moment that ranks as "worst." This apparent ambiguity

hy·po·der·mal

results from recognizing the stripes of damage caused by each "worst." My first worst had to do with the life-long physical destruction of all that was precious and the second worst came during the immediate emotional devastation caused by permanent separation. Shortly, I will share a third worst which injected a pain that has never ended. Time is said to heal all wounds. Let me tell you, that is pure malarkey. It may heal scratches and pokes, but when a major organ is ripped out of your chest, the wound may repair, but it never fully heals. At least not in this life.

This chopped version of my family took up residence with my father's sister and husband in the backwoods of Fosters, Alabama. I was left in the care of my aunt and I have very few recollections that are not horrible. For good or for bad, I was blessed with a remarkable memory and the bad memories are legion in this setting.

My aunt, or Knuckles, as I like to call her, believed sparing the rod was a mortal sin and a little chastening was pure love. In this regard, she loved the living stew out of me, employing thumb-thick switches on the backs of my bare legs, regularly and with enthusiasm.

I can't count the number of days I stood quivering and humiliated in my underwear sporting a fresh set of rising welts, knowing I had been convicted, but was absolutely innocent of any crime. Her favorite accusation was lying. I was guilty of many things, but lying was never a part of my nature.

As much as I hated my aunt for beating me, the fact that she rarely believed me was what forced me into silence and in that silence, I grew to despise her. There must have been days that were not bad, but I don't carry a single positive memory from my twelve-month century in Fosters.

As mean as Knuckles was, her husband terrified me. My father's brother-in-law was a monster. Over the years, in trying to investigate the events of that time, I was only able to garner a few faint recollections regarding my uncle from my father and brother.

I find it strange that neither I nor any of my family could recall a single specific memory, but I can say with absolute certainty, I felt endangered whenever I was alone with my uncle. Whatever he did, it must have been despicable and in my child's mind, he shadows me as the most horrible man in the world, my real-life boogeyman.

Dad was working long hours and my brother, who was now thirteen, spent his weekdays in school. Knuckles wouldn't let me watch television or remain indoors, forcing me to while away each day, entertaining myself without a single playmate or toy. I played with rocks, sticks and if I was very fortunate, a cardboard box. I had no idea who John Kennedy was at the time, but I can tell you with absolute certainty, I spent that entire day outside in a lonely yard the day he was assassinated. This was a miserable atmosphere in which to plunge a little boy who had just been ripped from his mother.

It is a blessing that five-year-olds are pretty much incapable of considering the future. I have endured a great deal of suffering from the anticipation of some unpleasant event or expected outcome. At this tender age, I greeted each day independently, with no comprehension that I had months of the same dreary torture and terror ahead of me. A single day was wretched enough without having to dread the next and the next.

If I had been capable of understanding and anticipating what my circumstances were, I would have sunk into despair and hopelessness. I suppose that is one of the reasons suicide rates remain low among the very young. Suicide requires despair and hopelessness and it takes a lot of evil adult behavior to drag a little one to that point.

Between the whippings, the loneliness, the boredom, the loss of my mother, and the terror of a monster, it is a miracle that I kept looking for any kind of good in my life. My father

hy·po·der·mal

did all he could and he was my only bright spot. I truly lived for the moment Dad came home from work.

I am sorry to say I don't have any positive recollections of my brother, although he may have played a more supportive role than I can remember. In my young mind, he was as much of a problem as everyone else in my life.

Oh, I almost forgot, I did have one friend during this solitary time, Brownie. That wonderful dog was my only companion and I still tear up with warm feelings for his loyalty so many decades ago. Right up until Brownie died in 1969, he did every bit as much to keep me sane as my father did. Animals can be an incredible positive influence for those of us struggling against depression.

Dad was struggling to learn the electrical trade, working as a helper for a contractor in Tuscaloosa. He once told me he was earning $1.25 per hour and that was why it took an entire year for him to gather enough money for us to flee Fosters and rent half a house in Tuscaloosa.

The rent of our new quarters was $40 per month and that provided us with a living room, dining room, bathroom, and a kitchen. Notice we had no bedrooms. For the next three years, Dad and I shared a bed in the dining room and my brother and Brownie shared a bed in the living room.

I doubt we had 300 square feet in which to live. It didn't matter to me that we were living right on the edge of poverty, as being away from Knuckles and Company was such a tremendous relief that even decades later I can still recall the feeling of joy and relief as we put that horrible house in our review mirror. I have never been incarcerated, but I have more than just an inkling of what being imprisoned and paroled must feel like.

This was 1964 and the only person available to watch out for six-year-old me was my brother. Once again, he may have done more for me than I remember, but if he was around very often, I have little or no recollection of it. My

hy·po·der·mal

few memories of him involve what is probably typical big brother behavior, making a little brother miserable.

During the summers, weekends, and after school, I was left to my own devices much as I had been in Fosters, but at least this time there were other children around and I was allowed to watch television (two whole channels!). I loved school and took to it very well, although my report cards are filled with requests for Dad to meet with my various teachers to address my behavior. The truth was that if any adult ever gave me a kind word, I would do backflips to deserve it. I just didn't get many kind words.

In October of 1965, I received the greatest joy I have ever felt. I also received my third and most devastating "worst." These two extremes occurred only forty-eight hours apart when my mother came to Alabama to do something. I got mixed reports on exactly what it was she wanted to accomplish, but whatever it was, it resulted in damaging me beyond my ability to fully repair – at least so far.

If you think about it, the difference between how a four-year-old and a seven-year-old processes information is immense. In fact, it is so profoundly different that it is practically the variance between an animal and a human. I say this to point out that I had experienced almost every one of my memories between the two and a half years I had been separated from my mother and the day she appeared on my porch. A relatively short time had passed for her, but for all intents and purposes, it felt like I had lived my entire life without a mother.

On that autumn afternoon, a strange woman knocked at my door shortly after I arrived home from school. I stood there, staring at her through the screen without the least clue as to who was standing in front of me. My blank look must have puzzled her. She asked me, "Don't you know who I am?" I told her I didn't. She said, "I'm your mother."

hy·po·der·mal

Can you imagine the explosion in my mind? I will never forget the joy of that moment. There may come a day when something overwhelms me as much as those three words did, but I have yet to imagine it. I had moved on and accepted life as it was, never expecting anything to change. I was motherless and yet miracle of miracles, I had a mother again.

Mom stayed for just two short days, although she later told me she had been in Tuscaloosa for a week. Whatever she hoped to accomplish with my father did not work out the way she wanted. I don't know what had ensued in her life from the time we drove away from her sister's porch, but apparently she had eventually moved in with the man with whom she'd had the affair, who had relocated to Chicago. Sometime during her visit, she secretly convinced my brother to return to Illinois with her, making promises that were never fulfilled.

Here comes "worst" number three. The day she and my brother left to return to Chicago was the greatest anguish I have ever felt. By far. To have regained a mother and then for her to once again reject me while stealing away my brother was more pain than my heart could take. It may have kept beating, but it shattered never to fully recover.

Mom wouldn't let me stay to see them off and insisted I leave the waiting room before she and my brother left. I stumbled out of the lobby and started the long walk home by myself. I remember a brilliant blue sky, but I was blind. I wept all the way home, my eyes finally running dry just as I walked into an empty house. I had never suffered like this before and as reality buried me, I felt all life drain away. As far as I was concerned, my mother had just rejected me and then died. For the first time (and not for the last time), I wondered if I shouldn't be dead as well.

I was a big fan of comic book Superman during this time. The Man of Steel had the capability of flying so fast that he could travel back in time and change events. Before all hope faded, I began to search for this ability in myself.

hy·po·der·mal

One day I explained to Dad what I would do if I could, thinking he would consider my time reversal plan a great idea. Much to my surprise, he told me that even if I could reverse time, he and my mother would never be together again. The second he said those words, all hope died and never returned.

About nine years later, I learned my mother had become pregnant with her third son only three months after abandoning me for the second time. I was not told of my younger half-brother for many years and didn't see my mother again until the day I graduated high school.

My older brother did not have a good experience with our mother in Chicago and after two years, returned to Alabama to enroll as a high school senior. One of the oddest quirks of this time was the fact that neither my brother nor I ever had a picture of our mother. It still took a while, but having no visual reminder made it a little easier to eventually exorcize her from my life. I had to, the pain was too great.

My father was smart, but he was not perfect. He told me many awful, but completely true things about my mother that should have never been spoken out loud to a young boy. He explained many of her very worst attributes, never saying anything positive. I was told time and again that my mother was untrustworthy and had not wanted my brother or me. It didn't take much to convince me.

I don't judge my father harshly for telling me these things. In his own way, he believed my mother was a toxic and deadly creature and he was doing all he could to make sure I severed every physical, mental, and emotional thread. Nevertheless, there is no doubt those words caused more damage than just about anything else ever said to me. Even if it is true, it is a dreadful thing to tell a child they are not wanted by a parent and the repercussions are inevitable and will always be dire. Some truths are not meant to be spoken, or at least they are not meant to be heard by little ears.

hy·po·der·mal

If there is ever a good time to be emotionally and physically severed from one's mother, I am certain it is not between the ages of four and seven. In fact, I have come to believe that is the worst possible time. During those tender years, nothing is complex, everything is divided and categorized as black and white and the idea of infinite shading is still below the horizon.

Additionally, each and every event is new and unique with memories sinking deep into the fertile ground of a young mind, some remaining as lively as can be and some to lie dormant for years to come. In other words, memories created during this formative period lay the foundation of our future thinking, they prejudice our minds.

I suspect it takes a lifetime of revelations, therapy, logic, and all sorts of adult interventions and insights for the full effect of certain memories to come to light. It is clear some terrors lurk buried behind walls and yet their existence is evidenced by behavior that can be explained in no other way. It is my belief that each of us becomes who we are during those early, developmental years. I don't mean to imply that we don't change and evolve, it is just that in my own experience, I have continued to bump into the same abandoned little boy regardless of my increasing maturation and understanding.

Years later, I came to realize that the same little boy had popped up unexpectedly many times throughout my young life, but the first time I recognized him, the experience frightened me. I was twenty-five and visiting my mother for only the second time. Things had been going very well up until she chose to make a small criticism regarding my older brother. All she said was a passing comment about how poorly he pitched-in around the house to help his wife. A large group of our family was sitting comfortably in my mother's living room when suddenly a viciousness exploded out of me that scared everyone, including myself.

hy·po·der·mal

Apparently, a perfect storm had been secretly brewing, collecting its energy, quietly and unseen. There were many feeders for this storm. My mother was still married to the man who helped destroy my own family and I was fully aware my resentment lie just below the surface, but I felt I was holding it in check.

My brother is a kind person and probably one of the most thoughtful and giving adults I have ever known and this makes me very defensive about him, a condition I have had all my adult life. Additionally, my brother has a non-aggressive demeanor and never fights back. Because of this character trait, there have been times when I have insinuated myself between him and his alleged assailant, often unwanted and always with disastrous results.

By this time in my life, I had developed a fairly calm and accepting disposition, but I possessed two ultra-hot buttons, betrayal and harming the innocent. Triggering either of these has and still can bring out primal responses from me. My mother, who had evolved into a cynical and complaining type, picked the wrong circumstances in which to belittle my brother.

The storm hit with blinding speed and an overwhelming anger vomited out of me, stunning everyone into silence. I was shaking with fury and the silence probably saved me from further trouble. I could have easily attacked the first person who gave me an excuse.

Obviously, an insult such as not helping with the dishes doesn't deserve such an over-the-top reaction. I was as surprised as anyone at the monster in the room. It was not pretty. Later, I pondered what had happened and for the first time, I realized there was still a damaged little boy inside me, raging and hurting, wanting to lash out at the woman who had abandoned and betrayed him. That had been trigger one.

The compounding trigger came by picking on my brother, a man who I felt deserved only kindness and appreciation for all he does. He was not perfect, but when it came to service he was a very good example to me. He qualifies as an innocent in my book.

Of course, I apologized and once I knew what had been silently building inside me, I was more careful to try to keep it under guard. In some ways, I was glad to learn the little boy was still with me. There had been lots of moments up to that point in my life in which I had overreacted inexplicably to some supposed offense, coincidentally involving some form of betrayal or an attack on the innocent. I finally had an explanation for these bewildering urges.

Given enough time, I figured I could eliminate my rage, but that was not going to happen. I have discovered it never really goes away and that I have to be vigilant to maintain control, especially in volatile situations involving trust. If you think about it, it is hard to be betrayed by someone you don't trust and that mostly leaves those who are closest and most influential in your life to take the brunt of your anger.

I have now spent six decades with that damaged little boy. It is always amazing to me that even though I add some increased comprehension of an important principle such as mercy or kindness, I continue to carry the same scarred four-year-old inside, just waiting to throw a tantrum of some sort.

One of my greatest mistakes over the years was trying to make the little boy go away. I thought knowledge and wisdom would make this possible. It is not. He is always there and will always be with me. What I have learned to do is work with him while increasing my understanding and kindness so that the tantrums grow fewer and reduce in magnitude.

From time to time, I have mistakenly thought I was doing a great job at controlling my urges and then, out of the blue, another perfect storm hits and the monster is unleashed. In no way am I trying to excuse my bad behavior, after all, I am the same person as the little boy. I am just trying to explain what is at the root of my bad behavior.

hy·po·der·mal

In order to understand my thinking, it may be necessary to slightly explain some of the common aspects of betrayal. We all have expectations for each other and each of us will fail in some manner those expectations. This is perfectly normal, human behavior. I think most people are pretty good at reacting to failed expectations with appropriate responses. It seems I have more trouble than most and I have come to believe part of the reason is rooted in being betrayed by my mother. She did not meet my expectations of what a mother should be.

I confess, I used to laugh at that sort of psychological mumbo jumbo, but no longer. From a seven-year-old's perspective, not only did she leave me, but she did it twice and the second time she took her "good" son with her and left behind the "bad" son. Couple with this the fact that my only trusted influence, my father, convinced me that my mother never wanted me and you can see how I might become deeply influenced by any act of betrayal.

I grew up in a time when everyone in my world (no exaggeration) had a mother in the home. This ate at me and reminded me of my worthlessness. Additionally, the women who I knew at school and church, almost certainly inadvertently, added to my feelings of worthlessness. As far as I could tell, no woman appeared to want much of anything positive to do with me, yet those same women all seemed to provide plenty of positive attention to my peers. I could add two and two as well as the next kid.

With my proven multi-rejections and now with what I experienced every day, what else could I conclude but that I was bad? The more other little boys received hugs and affection, the more attention I craved and the worse I behaved, leading to ever increasing negative responses. I grew to distrust women, after all, they treated me differently from other boys, and a deep prejudice was full-blown by the time I was eight years old.

hy·po·der·mal

Much of the bad behavior that follows throughout my life stems from angry responses to perceived betrayals – real or imagined really made no difference. No one could have known the far reaching effects that my mother's decision to destroy our family would have on me. My father could not have guessed what would happen when he told me my mother never wanted me. Who could have anticipated what taking my brother away and casting me aside a second time would reap down the road? I am still learning what role these things play in my life.

Your personal triggers may not have a thing to do with betrayal or protecting the innocent. Maybe you are fortunate enough to have no triggers at all. However, if you feel oppressed or discomfited, you most likely should at least consider what may have been planted deeply in your own young or not so young soul. When you react to something and then feel badly about it, you have just experienced a trigger. Triggers always make you sad. Know that there will be at least one root cause associated with it and uncovering the root is essential.

Just like my father, maybe the people sowing bad seeds had not the least intention of doing so, but that doesn't prevent the consequences of their actions. It is really hard to fix something when you only address symptoms. Finding the root cause is necessary if you want to make lasting change. If you are rolling your eyes, it's okay. I did too until I learned the value of such an effort. It is far more important than I could have guessed, but then again I used to be a raging skeptic of such things.

It may not be a good method for you, but I finally uncovered some of my root causes by writing. I tried therapists of all flavors and stripes, but must have only met the stupid ones. You may find a smart one and if you do, hang on and enjoy the ride. Just make sure they are not merely good guessers.

hy·po·der·mal

Maybe it will take a brutally honest and trusted friend or even an enemy to help you along your path. It is work, hard work, but it is worth every second. If you choose to write down your thoughts, the only thing that matters is that you never lie or mask the truth from yourself. Be brutally truthful, it is the only way to break through your natural defenses.

I don't know how to say this so that you can believe it, but there is a way for everyone to uncover enough truth to make a difference. Since I spent decades living, revering, and embracing a pack of self-imposed lies, I am proof of this. Some things are a fact and it is a fact that it doesn't take much at all to get the ball rolling. Just a tiny push and that will be enough. A little bit of truth, like a lit match in a dark cavern, goes a long way.

Your match in the darkness could just be a matter of pondering and producing questions about yourself with a trusted person or maybe even reading a book like this one might help. None of us are so unique that we can't learn some truth from one another. Even your worst enemy can (and often does) reveal important, previously hidden essentials. Mine sure did.

I have never been accused of being overly bright, but through sheer doggedness and perseverance, I found five unshakable truths – albeit they came just as my hope was choking on life-support. I won't speak of these just yet because unshakable truths seem to come best in layers, line upon line so to speak. The next chapter continues our journey of root exposure during which a few more layers of gunk and even some truth may appear. Keep your eyes open for it.

What I Just Tried to Say, but in Fewer Words

- Root causes are the beginnings and drivers of all the self-inflicted problems in our lives.

hy·po·der·mal

- The mind really can make a heaven out of hell or a hell out of heaven, but not when it is confused.
- Root Causes must be exposed before you can make lasting changes. We spend an inordinate amount of time treating symptoms.
- Root Causes will never leave, but their effects are controllable.
- Triggers are things can lie hidden for years and yet ironically, their symptoms can manifest all day long, every day. We see their effect, but often don't understand the underlying cause. Triggers always make us sad.
- Enforcers are those events that pound triggers into your soul. Examples might include indifferent teachers or a mistaken, but well-meaning father. They are destructive by anyone's definition, but not necessarily intentionally so. Surprisingly, enforcers are easy to spot, just follow the path to the cause of your pain.

P.S. Please don't judge my mother harshly. There is no question that she made terrible choices, but what is not apparent are the terrible root causes in her own life. She was abused by her father, brothers, and her brother's friends and spent many days of her childhood hiding in cornfields in order to survive. No one but her knows what triggers were being pulled during this period in my young life. I do not feel qualified to judge her motivations, but that doesn't release me from the consequences of her actions, it only begs for us to be merciful, which is something we all could use.

hy·po·der·mal

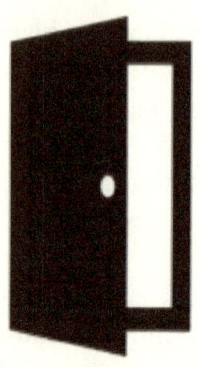

in·flu·ence

    I often wished a lady, any lady, would hug me, but none of my school or church teachers ever felt inclined to do so. Women gradually became increasingly foreign to me. Other than my mother, I don't remember ever being hugged by a woman until the summer I turned nine-years-old. The act was so rare, that I can still recall the time of day and location where it happened.
    Probably related to this, I was the kid everyone hated in their class, the noisy boy constantly acting up for attention. To their credit, none of my teachers ever seemed to become overly angry, but to their shame, none ever gave me the love I was seeking either.
    Some may say it is not a teacher's job to provide love, but I believe with every fiber of my being it is the only job worth doing and teaching is ancillary at best, at least it was in my particular situation. I can say this with some authority because I have spent more than four decades teaching children and the appropriate and discrete application of love in the classroom, or any setting for that matter, augments and often trumps teaching every time.
    I had been torn to pieces by the betrayals of my mother, a misguided aunt and uncle, and the neglect of each woman

who could have added a touch of kindness to my life. I was searching for someone to fill the gaps, but all I can remember are punishments or at best, indifference.

Of course, the more I was disciplined for my attention-seeking behavior, the greater the hunger for what I was missing. There finally came a point where I concluded bad attention was better than no attention. It was truly a miracle that I did not develop into a sociopath. The few times some woman, almost always a stranger, would say or do some kind thing, it seemed to impact me profoundly. A kind word or a compliment was water in my desert, very rare, but oh so greatly appreciated.

My fourth grade teacher was the sole exception of my youth and she may have single-handedly prevented me from heading down a very dark path. Early on, I discovered she had a sympathetic ear and I honestly thought I was manipulating her just for attention. I felt guilty about my actions, but I was starving. She would take me out into the hall so we could speak privately. Mostly I cried, often crocodile tears, as she intently listened to what I said and what I didn't say.

I contacted this sainted woman some fifty years later and she remembered me very well. Needless to say, I was shocked. It turns out she knew all along I had been playing on her sympathy, but she realized that I actually needed love and allowed me to "use" her as often as I felt the need to do so. If there ever was a defining example of true religion among us mortals, she was one.

At the other end of the spectrum was my grade school principal. He had a lot of people fooled, but I had learned to recognize monsters early on from my uncle and this man was one. I tried to stay off his radar, but my crying-talks out in the hall set me in his sights early and I stayed there for the next three years. Like so many of his ilk, this man should have never been allowed anywhere near children.

hy·po·der·mal

Out on the playground, he would often join the boys in football, playing quarterback for both teams. He always had me hike the ball to him and then my job was to run a few steps, turn sharply around and wait for a pass. He was a big man and could throw the ball very hard. Keep in mind that I was only a few feet away from him and I dreaded the moment he decided I was his target.

I will never forget the look in his eyes and the way he would grit his teeth when he would wind-up and throw with all his might, trying to knock me down. I was a stubborn kid and I never dodged his passes. Most would hammer me to the ground or bounce painfully off my chest, but every now and then I hung onto one. Those were great victories in my mind.

Many children are predisposed to selfishness or self-centeredness, but under the circumstances, I was doomed to push the extremes. Having little reason to learn selflessness or to put another's needs before my own, I simply became more and more unpleasant. My boundary-pushing behavior set up a vicious cycle in which it became increasingly difficult for me to make friends.

I was fortunate that a few boys liked to spend time with me despite my flawed character and a couple of these childhood friends possessed unusually good character traits which I found myself coveting. I really didn't have the tools to change myself, but I genuinely wanted to be a nicer person because of the good boys around me. My heart may have been damaged, but it was still a good one.

The year I spent as a nine-year-old was pivotal in a number of ways. We moved from our half of house in the city to a small, two-bedroom home located deep in the woods of the county. This meant a return to my familiar isolated way of life. During the seven years I lived there, I was never well-accepted by any of the established families surrounding my neck of the woods, none of whom lived within shouting distance of my house.

hy·po·der·mal

For an area so sparsely populated, it was quite amazing that I ended up encircled by twelve similarly aged boys within a two mile radius of my home. Sadly, only one of these boys ever considered me a good friend, with the rest rotating from mild adversaries to violent enemies depending on what openings were available.

I don't know if I brought these conflicts on myself due to my selfish nature or if it was the circumstance of being the new city boy intruding among country people who had resided in the area for decades or even centuries. I do know I was the only one without a mother among my peers and that I spent countless days either alone or dodging bullies.

I had two major influences for good at this time. One was a boy who shared my next three grade school classes and one was a boy who became my best friend at church. I am very grateful to have fallen under their combined influence.

The boy at school was one of the most unlikely of people to have played the role he did. He was a social misfit who had already failed one grade. This boy did me two great favors. First, he introduced the game of football to me. This was my initial exposure to "grown-up" sports. I went on to fall in love with all manner of athletics, ranging from badminton to rugby, and even though I put my heart and soul into each and every one, football was the only one that made my heart soar. I loved being a part of a team.

Second, this boy could draw. I liked drawing and although I was creative, I was limited to a very rudimentary skill set. This kid could reproduce three-dimensional, life-like masterpieces and displayed a vast talent. I copied everything he did, practiced at home, and wasted many hours trying to convince others I was more capable than my Example. Everyone, including me, knew my self-imposed contests were never even close.

True to my self-absorbed nature and even though I owed this boy a tremendous debt, I never treated him well and went out of my way to demean him behind his back. It took nearly forty years for me to get around to apologizing and thanking him for the wonderful influence he had been. Amazingly, he only remembered me as a good friend.

The other powerful influence in my childhood was an unusually good-hearted and very, very smart boy. He read and studied everything he could get his hands on, while I was still flipping comic book pages. He studied religious writings, Sherlock Holmes, cryptography, and dozens of other fields of knowledge normally reserved for more mature audiences.

I found myself fascinated by the things he introduced to me. We attended church together and I was stunned to find someone my age that didn't resent attending meetings or reading books of scripture. I couldn't believe it when he admitted he did these things of his own volition.

I was jealous of him, but he was so kind-hearted that I could barely stand to constantly and consistently put him down. Despite my rotten treatment, he never gave up on me and eventually taught me to be less selfish.

The two of us have stayed in touch and from time to time we have met and chatted as old friends. Long ago, I recognized the debt owed him and still regularly express my gratitude. He not only influenced me with good morals, but his studious nature built in me a desire to excel in my schoolwork. Of course, I had the competing desire to take shortcuts and only perform to minimum standards, but between these extremes, I managed to become a better than average student in spite of myself.

Both of these boys were incredibly important because I was never able to hit any sort of social mainstream until high school. Without their help, I fear I would have sought ever descending levels of societal behavior.

All through grade school and junior high, it seemed any friend I had was my friend because I worked at it, not once was it the other way around. I don't know, maybe most of

hy·po·der·mal

us feel that way, but one thing I can say for certain, I suffered through thousands of lonely hours when I would have much rather been spending time with a friend or even a semi-friendly antagonist.

I can't explain why, but none of the boys living around me ever wanted to come to my house. Not once in seven years. I spent many days wandering the hour-long circuit between houses, hoping to find someone who would play with me. All too often, I returned home to watch our two-channel television set or bounce a ball off the carport wall.

Out of desperation, I concocted a schizophrenic form of playing board games, cards, and even played chess against myself. Pretending I was two different people, I consciously blocked thoughts so that I would not anticipate what the other me's next move would be. Sometimes I picked sides against myself and would get frustrated when the wrong me would lose.

It didn't help that I was grossly lacking in the social graces. Goodness knows my father did the best he could, but I think we were probably living barely above a savage state. I know for a fact that we never cleaned our bathroom, I rarely had a toothbrush, and I set a personal ten-year-old record of going two weeks without bathing.

The few times I was invited to visit someone's home, inevitably something embarrassing would be repeated back to me by my chum. The only time I ate dinner at a classmate's home I was later told the adults had referred to me as the "little boy who wouldn't stop talking." This sort of feedback didn't do much for my self-esteem.

Even as a pre-teen, I had a ton of anger issues. I was angry with my circumstances in life, my loneliness, my lack of friends, and for who knows how many other reasons. Generally, I didn't seek fights, but I sure didn't try very hard to avoid them either. Sometimes I would swap punches and sometimes I would just scream out my aggravation. I wasn't a bad boy, I was just frustrated with perceived injustices and

hy·po·der·mal

when I felt one of my triggers surge through me I could become a proverbial honey badger.

Adults were not off limits to me. As a young teenager, I once grew to despise a man who happened to be my scoutmaster and although he was six-feet two, a retired fighter pilot, outweighed me by a hundred pounds and twenty-five years my senior, my triggers knew no boundaries. He had a snide and arrogant way of making others feel inferior and I was his target more often than all my fellow scouts combined. I don't think he had the foggiest idea that he was bullying a boy with deep resentments just waiting for a chance to release them.

One night, after another verbal evisceration, I finally reacted, threatening him and calling him a coward for picking on children. This happened in front of the entire troop and even those who knew my capabilities, were astonished. This man was in his second year of law school at the time and I think he realized that he could go to prison for taking the bait and managed to keep his cool. We were never best friends and he later publicly humiliated me in a scouting review board as payback. As bad as he was, I was actually surprised when he was exposed as a sexual predator by his daughter.

The loneliness that I experienced as a young country boy wasn't nearly as miserable as what I had endured trapped at my aunt's house. That had been much more prison-like. During my country days, the second of what will be four isolated periods in my life (two in my youth and two in my golden years), things were considerably better in that I could read, had access to television, and possessed some toys and balls to add variety to my day. Maybe this is a kind of loneliness that many children experience, particularly those who are isolated by geography.

In the summer of 1972, my father decided to remarry. I was fourteen years old and resented this intrusion into our bachelor-way-of-life. The woman he brought into our house

hy·po·der·mal

was deaf and had not the least clue of how to deal with a teenager – even though I happened to be one of the less rebellious types. None of us gave it much thought, but in retrospect it would have been useful to check with me on this decision if only to find out what alligators were hiding in my swamp. There were lots and they were a moody sort.

Not only did I have my general resentment for women, but we couldn't help but have communication difficulties. Under normal circumstances, the two of us would have butted heads, but her deafness made our hurdles monumental. It didn't help matters that she was in her fifties when we first met. That fact alone meant we looked at the world from conflictive perspectives. Not surprisingly, our relationship started poorly, went downhill, and eventually plunged over a cliff ending in a modest nuclear detonation.

I made some choices that were simply stupid. The worst of them was that once she and her furniture had shoehorned into our house, I figured what was hers was now mine. I think I vaguely understood the concept of privacy, but I still rooted through her stuff, taking whatever I wanted. As you might imagine, she was not thrilled with my actions. Friction began to increase and neither of us had sufficient skills to address any topic, shallow or deep. On top of that, she wanted the bathroom kept clean.

My new step-mother had to use a special device on our single phone that amplified both sides of a conversation, making everything easily overheard. I made it a point to go to my room as she spent hours talking with old friends about her difficulties, some of which I assume included me. To my credit, once I was in my room, I shut my door, turned up some music, and made it a point to never listen in. I understood privacy very well in that regard.

One night my father, in an utterly sincere but horribly misguided attempt at working out our difficulties, gathered us into the living room to voice our grievances. He chose a round-robin format and his new wife was asked to begin. It

hy·po·der·mal

is a genuine tragedy that I wasn't asked to start, because I was going to say that I was sorry for being inconsiderate and that I would try to do better. What a difference that night might have seen had I gone first. This is one of those big "might have beens."

The poor lady's opening words accused me of the one thing I had gone out of my way to respect, declaring her disgust that I had been eavesdropping on her phone calls. I was guilty of so much, why on earth had she zeroed in on the one thing for which I was innocent? Keep in mind my triggers regarding betrayal and attack of the innocent were always lying just barely below the surface.

As a fourteen-year-old, I had plenty of normal issues, but I also had a couple that were highly abnormal. I am not talking about common teen-age angst, selfish behavior, or pride, but an intense resentment of any womanly intrusion. The very fact that once again another woman had proved to be an adversary rather than a friend would have put me in a bad state and the honest truth was that my expectations had been perfectly formed for failure. I had expected a loving, caring mother and had ended up with anything but that. Betrayal and Innocence! Of course, I exploded.

Years of pent-up anger came boiling out with a laser focus on this tiny, deaf creature who had just wrongly accused me. I raged out of control. She was terrified and leaped from her chair, screaming, "That boy is going to kill me!" Frightened for her life, she fled the house, jumped in her car, and stayed far away for several days. I was delighted, but my father was crushed.

Of course, I now realize she had her own challenges in trying to adjust to marriage after being single for over half her adult life. She had given up a familiar world in Birmingham and moved-in with a couple of hillbillies in backwards Northport, Alabama. Once she returned to our home, the two of us hardly ever spoke to each other again.

hy·po·der·mal

It was an incredibly miserable situation and I never felt secure and I am sure she felt the same.

Three years later, I left for college and was forbidden to ever return to my home again. I couldn't help but feel my father had betrayed me as well at that point. He had made his choice and I was the loser once more. Now, nobody wanted me.

Oddly, even though I resented the situation, I understood that my father had done about the best he could, since I was due to be leaving the nest anyway and his wife desperately needed both his support and my disappearance. On some level, I understood what he was doing and why he was doing it, but logic and reason don't always prevail when it comes to deeply rooted emotions. Given my track record, I was forced to conclude I was no good.

Some forty years later, shortly before my antagonist died, she referred to herself as my "evil step-mother" in a witty and well-received speech at a family reunion. Even I laughed. She had a son, several years older than me, who was a very tender-hearted soul. He spoke privately with his mother sometime during that reunion, telling her that she knew she had treated me cruelly and that she also knew she could do better.

He later shared with me she had agreed with him, but then had added, "But not in this life." She died in 2011, having spoken only a handful of words to me over the years. I had made dozens of heart-felt attempts to repair the alienation caused by my fourteen-year-old anger, but just like her, I found it was not to be in this life.

What I Just Tried to Say, but in Fewer Words

- You don't always get to pick who influences you. If you think little children are not powerfully influenced by peers, you need to think a little harder.

hy·po·der·mal

- Bad little boys (and little girls) are not bad, they just need more love than they are getting.
- Expectations are essential and not having expectations is dumb. However, attaching your emotions to your expectations is very dumb and will lead you into a world of hurt.
- Everyone, including yourself is guaranteed to fail and fall short of your expectations some of the time. That is the very definition of being human and I believe it is the purpose of life, otherwise why not just watch the video?

hy·po·der·mal

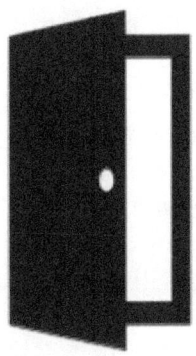

com·mit·ment

Until I entered high school, I had zero girlfriends and this was completely by choice, just not mine. Whatever attribute boys with girlfriends possessed, I was missing just about one hundred percent of it. If you take into account my feelings of betrayal regarding women, it is not much of a stretch to assume this condition did not help matters and likely served to further cement my mistrust.

My non-girlfriend status wasn't from a lack of trying either. I stuck my neck out into the treacherous and humiliating interplay between boys and girls many times, but relentless rejections gradually moved me into a protective shell, smothering my feelings and hopes. This is a perfect example of an unintentional, but no less deadly, enforcer on my triggers.

I would have welcomed any kind of positive attention from the opposite sex, but it wasn't until I was sixteen years old that I was finally coaxed out of my shell. Up until that time, I honestly wondered what was wrong with me and if it hadn't been for a wonderful girl in my high school junior year, there was probably some sort of hermitage in my future.

hy·po·der·mal

Just to ram home the thought of how naïve I was, as a sixteen-year-old, I once asked a girl-acquaintance if kissing involved one lip or two. I never forgot the peculiar look I received. Believe me, I was perfectly groomed to be a recluse.

My first girlfriend knocked off a ton of my rough edges and for all the happiness I experienced in her company, the friendship was eventually obliterated by an as yet undisclosed fault deeply hidden in my character. Symptoms had manifest before that time, but remained incomprehensible until an epiphany will rip open and exposed the surprising flaw some four decades later. I will carry a massive and unnecessary grief for an awful long time, but more on that in a bit.

This girl was someone with whom I had once spent a few hours at a church youth gathering some eighteen months earlier. She was a year older than me and I had just turned fifteen at the time. This meant she was sixteen and driving and that made all the difference in terms of anything beyond being an acquaintance. We danced a few dances and things ended with no hint of any future contact – not my choice, definitely hers. I chalked up another successful failure.

A year and a half later, while wall-flowering a New Year's Eve dance, I bumped into my old friend and I asked her if she'd like to dance. We wobbled back and forth, talking about what had changed in our lives and then, as the song ended and I prepared to return to my wall-support duties again, the most astonishing thing happened. Someone grabbed my hand and held it and as I investigated, I could see it was a hand belonging to the girl.

To someone who had never had any sort of contact other than the casual and superficial kind, this was earthshattering. I love hyperbole as much as the next fellow, but I was honestly stunned that a girl was holding my hand and have never forgotten the thrill that raced through me. I have never taken an illicit drug or ingested any alcohol, but if that is the

hy·po·der·mal

kind of feeling that can result, I can certainly understand the attraction.

I didn't have a clue what this interdigitation meant and frankly, I didn't care. The very fact that someone wanted to hold my hand stands as the highpoint of my teen years and one of the happiest moments of my life. Even though we lived sixty miles apart, we ended up dating until she left for college and as far as I was concerned, it was a perfect relationship. She was witty, morally focused, and understood what teen dating was all about. She was much more mature than me and raised the bar for my behavior by several notches while teaching me important dating etiquette rules such as quart applications of cologne were not necessary. Most importantly, I learned to be a gentleman under her tutelage.

We spent all our time together doing fun, creative things and other than sitting close or holding hands, there was not even a hint of any romance. I learned more about how to communicate effectively and how to think of the other person's point of view from this girl than almost any other person in my life. She taught me how to create a relationship first with my mind, delaying other aspects until the right time and circumstances.

When she left to attend an out of state school, I would have continued our relationship to whatever degree and in whatever fashion she would've allowed, but she simply dropped me. Sadly, but not unexpectedly, I interpreted this behavior as not only rejection, but also betrayal.

The very fact that she was the first girl to ever want my company was enough motivation in my acceptance-starved life for me to stick by her side forever. If she had wanted to stay in touch by phone or correspondence, I would have done so as long as it took until we were reunited.

One of my most enduring qualities is loyalty and I was more than prepared to be loyal to her as we married and grew old together. I realize that my viewpoint was naïve and

hy·po·der·mal

immature, but it was absolutely sincere nonetheless. Keep in mind, I had never, not even once, had a girl indicate that she wanted to spend any sort of exclusive time with me. I figured this was a once in a lifetime occurrence for a fellow like me and even though my understanding was warped, I was genuinely willing to commit for life.

It stung, but I managed to survive this rejection and even had a fragile hope that there might be some other girl out there who could find me interesting. I started my senior year and having now been in a dating relationship, I was slightly less fearful when approaching girls. The first day of school I chatted with a girl who I thought might have some potential, but if she had any interest in me, she was using words that appeared to mean just the opposite.

I gave it my all for a month, but ultimately out of sheer confusion and exhaustion, I stopped trying. By the time that misery came to an end, I had lost what little confidence I might have gained and sailed back into the relationship doldrums. I consciously and sincerely shut down all further social attempts and determined I would never date again.

During this time, a girl had taken a liking to me, but I was so wrapped up in my own failures that I never had a clue. We shared a math class and the two of us "happened" to be walking together to our next class. I found out later that some girls are wily and can be downright devious when they choose to be. This innocent-looking creature, casually asked me who I was taking to Homecoming. I flatly told her, "nobody," but distinctly remember thinking, "What am I supposed to do with a question like that?"

After a second or two of uncomfortable silence and in an attempt at pure politeness, I responded by asking her who was her date. Her answer surprised me. She said she wasn't going. I was completely oblivious to her smoothly delivered guile, although I probably wouldn't have recognized it even with a flashing neon sign.

hy·po·der·mal

Genuinely curious, I asked her, "Why not?" Again, her answer caught me off guard. She quietly said, "Because no one has asked me." I had never paid attention to her before and barely knew her name, but in a genuine moment of chivalry, I piped up and said I would be glad to take her, fully expecting my offer to be politely declined. With no hesitation she responded, "That would be great." It took several long seconds for me to understand that I had a date for Homecoming.

On the night of our first date, about everything that could go wrong did go wrong. I was the unwilling master of ceremonies for the halftime show during the homecoming game and was as nervous as I've ever been. I showed up late at my date's house because I hadn't bothered to ask where she lived. Her whole family was leaving and my car, which was parked blocking her driveway, wouldn't start. After casting chicken bones and chanting, I managed to get the engine running and by then we were so late, we were forced to park quite a distance away from the stadium.

As I got out of the car, I had the presence of mind to open her door, but then started mindlessly racing toward the stadium, not really noticing if my poor date could keep up. About forty feet from the car, while trotting down a dark alley, I was scared out of my skin as something unexpectedly grabbed my right hand. Stifling a scream, I looked down and it turned out to be my date's left hand. For the second time in my life I was surprised to find someone wanted to hold my hand. Here is another memory that stands as a top ten among my most joyful moments of life.

We ended up becoming the very best of friends and I spent as much time as I could around her. She was the most selfless and service-oriented person I had ever met. My admiration and love for her grew daily and from time to time, I spoke frankly to her of how our relationship would certainly continue and never end. To me, this way of thinking made perfect sense. I figured once you loved

hy·po·der·mal

someone, it was for life. We were both only seventeen years old and completely unknown to me, this girl had a different view of what her life would become.

We dated during the entire school year and I sailed through graduation blissfully content that I had found my soulmate. Early in the summer, she started dropping hints that our dating relationship was temporary. She was extremely tender with me and did everything within her power to let me down easily, but I was too blind to see what she was trying so very graciously and kindly to tell me. I just kept blathering on about our joined future.

Finally, there came a day when she was forced to explain to me that we were not going to date again, making it clear she wanted us to remain great friends. She was really smart and was probably not surprised to see I was totally unprepared for her emancipation. I immediately treated her kindness as a rejection. I felt betrayed again by the person I thought I would spend the rest of my life with and as has already been discussed, betrayal is not something that I handle well.

I severed the relationship altogether and my heart re-shattered. It is amazing to me that I silently and secretly carried the pain of this failure for the rest of my life. The intensity faded with time, but I never got over the fact that my soulmate had kicked me to the curb.

It wasn't until I was in my late fifties that I experienced the epiphany I referred to a few pages earlier and finally understood my teenage expectation had never been remotely the same as my girlfriend's. What I interpreted as rejection and betrayal had been nothing but perfectly normal behavior from a sweet, intelligent seventeen-year-old girl. In fact, if anything, she had performed quite brilliantly and maturely for such an innocent age. It took an awful long time, but I finally learned that she had never been my enemy, but had always been a true friend. What a waste.

hy·po·der·mal

However, at that time I found myself once again rejected. I was bad. I deserved rejection. I was a failure because I had wanted to commit for life to two girls and neither of them wanted me. Due to the roots buried so deep, no one could have known the way my mind worked until events will finally occur to expose my misunderstandings. There will be a lot of tears shed between that time and today.

At the right time and under the right circumstances, such a level of commitment can be a ferocious benefit, but the fact that I felt rejected, coupled with my lack of understanding, a deep and severe scarring developed that was totally unnecessary and self-inflicted. I felt I had offered all I had to give to each of my young loves and that had not been enough for them. I knew I had nothing left to offer and was left with the obvious and faulty conclusion that my best would always be inadequate.

Just like my mother and just like the other women, I had given my best and something else was wanted. I had no ability to recognize that my premature timing might have had anything to do with my circumstances. I really did see things simply and with my desperate need to be accepted, I had developed impossible expectations that could only have resulted in failure. I had no realistic path to success and how could I have guessed that it was my expectations that were faulty and not me? My offerings had seemed so noble and tragically, I won't understand how misguided they were for a very long time.

Obviously, I have now dropped enough hints to indicate something big is coming down the road. I am not playing teasing games with you. I hope you find the story interesting and there really is a method to my madness. What will happen that changed my life and has the potential to help others as well, needs to be understood through the experiences that precede the revelation.

Please be patient. In the meantime, try to spot those connections in your own life that are in no way identical to

hy·po·der·mal

my own, but involve similar principles and challenges. I have failed. You have failed. Let's see if we can take our failures and make something wonderful happen.

What I Just Tried to Say, but in Fewer Words

- Not only is hitching your love to an expectation bad for relationships, but if you happen to have picked an impossible expectation, there is zero chance of a positive outcome.
- The mismatches of life are probably just as important as the matches. This doesn't mean they are fun though. Lots of important stuff hurts like crazy.
- You may not have the same abnormal attribute I had of committing way beyond what is appropriate, but it is a good bet that you do have some attribute that is a little skewed. Take the time to examine your deepest pains and see if you too don't have something a little out of whack regarding your interpretation of events.

P.S. That wonderful, beautiful, incredible girl attempted suicide just a couple of years later for the very reasons I have written. She was driven to this action because she thought she had failed. She had actually chosen to link her happiness to an expectation that was never possible. She couldn't help but achieve an outcome that would disappoint her. She survived her attempt, but has lived the rest of her days institutionalized. I still grieve for her.

hy·po·der·mal

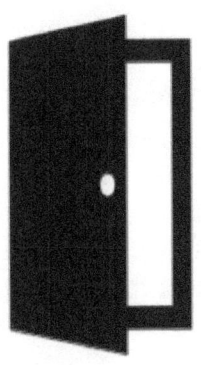

grasp·ing

Many years ago, I saved someone from drowning. It was a painful experience because the person was panicked out of his mind and trying to survive by any means, even if it meant killing his potential savior. Unbelievably, I rescued this fellow twice in one weekend. After all the clawing and kicking I had received from my first effort, I learned to keep my distance by diving below him and pushing him to safety. Watch out for those who are grasping for life, they desperately need your help and will eagerly help you into desperation. In this chapter, I am begin grasping.

Now that I was an unquestionable reject and the best I had to offer was unwanted by any female, I fell into a survival way of thinking and it was not particularly beneficial to my emotional well-being.

If I have been paying attention, I have now shared with you the root (abandonment and the need for acceptance) of my two triggers (betrayal and afflicting the innocent), a few of the enforcers (misguided adults and indifference from teachers and girls), and the added bonus attribute of unreal expectations through over-commitment (based on my desperate need for acceptance). Woo doggy, we are well along our path of uncovering some root causes of depression and suicide. Your life will most likely have totally different roots, but the process of uncovering will be very similar, possibly even identical. Stay with me, help is on the way.

I had no clue my expectations were faulty nor did I have a clue my willingness to commit went far beyond what might be considered anywhere near a normal progression between two people. I didn't have the foggiest idea that I was still seeking the acceptance that had been long lost at the beginning of my path. All I knew was that everywhere I turned, even though I was willing to give all that I had, nothing I offered was acceptable – or at least that is how I interpreted events. Betrayal. Betrayal. Betrayal.

Soon I will start looking for some sort of trick, shortcut, or even legitimate tool for success, but not for a few years yet. I still need to make a couple more spectacularly misdirected choices to finally corrupt all my thinking. I will do just that, but in the meantime, let's see what else can seem so right, but be so wrong.

As a college freshman, I tried a remarkable number of times to connect with any girl at school, despite a perfect string of rejections. In retrospect, I find myself admiring and pitying that young fellow who just wouldn't give up. That may have been one of the most disappointing yet bravest periods of my life. A few of my college failures were brutal, building resentment that sometimes manifest in vivid and humiliating outbursts directed at people not even involved. Little boy tantrums were alive and well.

Eventually, I gave up on searching among my peers and began seeking less risky relationships. I was eighteen and found a fourteen-year-old who I could spend time with. Please don't ascribe any untoward behavior in this. I was utterly innocent, had only high moral and perfectly decent intentions. There was not even a smidgeon of impropriety in such a relationship as far as I was concerned. I simply wanted a friend I could trust not to hurt me.

hy·po·der·mal

After a few weeks, my potential friend's mother made it crystal clear there was something wrong with me. Once again, I was completely caught off guard and confused by the woman's severe rejection. I had visited the girl a couple of times at her house, spent some afternoons skateboarding with her brother, and mowed their gigantic lawn a couple of times. I thought I had become a trusted friend of the family. After being told to never return, I got the message.

There had been hints for some time that a girl at church, three and a half years my junior, had expressed some interest in me. As a self-absorbed sixteen-year-old, I had been told this same girl, when twelve-years-old, had once said to a friend, "I'm going to wrap that boy (me) around my little finger someday." That sort of thing can be taken at least two ways. One, I could have been flattered or two, I could have been annoyed. I chose door number two and spent the next few years callously teasing the young girl. Not one of my prouder moments.

Coincidentally, my father liked this girl and one day he asked me to drive him some sixty miles to attend her piano recital in Birmingham. I had scuba diving plans for that weekend, but my father was a class-A wheedler and soon had me chauffeuring him for what I assumed would be a dreadful evening among doilies and grandmas. When I drove onto a university campus and parked outside of the main concert hall, I noticed a distinct lack of doilies.

The twelve-year-old girl had grown up considerably and looked very mature as a fifteen-year-old in a formal gown, walking across the stage under a bright spotlight. I was situated between her father and my own, and managed to not hate my first exposure to classical music.

As I sat, gaping around at the large audience, I remember clearly thinking that this girl used to like me and it might be possible to rekindle that feeling again. Maybe, just maybe, I could have her as a friend in spite of our age difference. At the concert end, a gaggle of boys walked on

hy·po·der·mal

stage to embrace her and hand her bouquets of roses. I decided then and there I would see if there was still a spark.

After the concert, my father and I were invited to her home for a reception. I spoke with her and chased away all the competition. Surprisingly, her parents were amenable to my developing some sort of friendship. In retrospect, I can't believe they let me, almost nineteen-years-old by this time, visit regularly with their daughter.

Some years later, the mother told me that both she and her husband had felt some concern at the time, but that she had made it a matter of prayer and said it had been made perfectly clear to her, "Not only was it alright, but it was necessary." I, of course, had no idea of these behind the scenes workings and just hoped I had found a friend who wouldn't reject me.

I look back on those halcyon days and knowing just how completely innocent I was, I can say without a doubt I had only the best interests of that young lady at heart. By this time, not only was I becoming skilled in gentlemanly manners, but I had shaken loose an astonishing amount of selfishness and become a genuinely kind-hearted person.

Nobody in this situation could have known that it was the fear of betrayal that was building and driving my need for this relationship. It was never a conscious thought, but years after the fact, I realized that I was in survival mode, figuring I could grasp onto someone who was so young, especially with the approval of her parents.

Speaking of her parents, this girl's mother stands as one of the brightest influences in my life. I was right on the cusp of becoming a man, just at that bridge between child and adult when she stepped in and did something no one else could have done – at the very last moment it could have been accomplished, she became a real mother to me.

This kind woman recognized what a desperate yearning I had for a mother's love and wrapped me up and accepted me for who I was. Had I been older, I could have never

hy·po·der·mal

allowed such a thing to happen, but I was just young enough to soak up this rare gift, the very one I had sought all my life. There was never any question that she genuinely loved me. She often said to me and to others that if her daughter and I did not stay connected, I would still always be her son. I believed her.

This form of love, a mother's love, probably accomplished more repair to my soul than I will ever be able to fully comprehend. I was well on the way to becoming a good person, but was dragging along some massive flaws and her generosity was miraculously effective at accelerating my good character traits while simultaneously reducing the ugly stuff. I had an innate desire to do good and to avoid bad and although her influence did not eliminate my self-destructive capabilities, she did give me some tools to lessen their impact and to repair the damage after the fact.

Not surprisingly, I once again assumed this budding friendship would lead to a lifelong relationship, after all, it seems I had a mother (in-law) long before I would have a spouse. Through the lens of time, I am embarrassed at my immaturity and childish way of thinking, but that is exactly where my thoughts were. I couldn't imagine that I would be rejected this time.

It never occurred to me that a fifteen-year-old girl might ever want to date anyone else and have other relationships now that she had the complete attention of someone so much older invested in her. I wasn't stupid, but I was naïve, assuming that we were soulmates and nothing would ever stop our destiny – regardless of the fact that things had not worked out that way for me, twice. Or then again, maybe I was stupid, but I'd like to think I was just foolishly optimistic. Regardless, I suspect I was too desperate for acceptance to allow myself to consider any other outcome.

The two of us spent most of what time we had together at her house from June to September of 1977. I think we only went on two dates. During the heart of the summer, she

hy·po·der·mal

and her family spent an entire month out of state. We lived sixty miles apart and after all was said and done, we actually only spent a total of twenty or so days together during the four months.

It is hard to believe that I built such a deep relationship in my mind on such a short time and under such odd circumstances. I turned nineteen, she was fifteen, and we really didn't have much of anything in common and couldn't date in any sort of normal fashion. By anyone's definition this was unusual.

In fact, it was considered very controversial by some of the nosey-nellies in the churches we attended, mine in Tuscaloosa and hers in Birmingham. We were both threatened by church leadership that we needed to cease our relationship or there might be consequences. Her family was ostracized to a minor degree.

These Romeo and Juliet circumstances may have been the glue that held the relationship together that summer. I suppose we were actually strengthened by those seeking to tear us apart. I don't ascribe any bad intentions to those who opposed us. I think most of them simply thought it was every bit as weird as it appeared to be. And it sure didn't help that there was a church-wide mandate that there should be no dating of any church member until the age of sixteen.

To anybody on the outside, it might have appeared we were dating like crazy, flagrantly denouncing all that was good and holy. Our time together was heavily chaperoned, although it was not necessary, but still welcome as far as I was concerned. I loved her mother and never regretted having her around. Technically, one of our two dates was in violation of the rules, but we were home not long after dark and the movie had been squeaky clean. The other date had been a double-date with her parents and that hardly counts.

We had entered this arrangement knowing there was a deadline in September. I had long planned on serving a two-year mission for my church when I turned nineteen and by

hy·po·der·mal

July I learned I was going to South Korea. Maybe that and the fact that I was about as good a boy as could be was why the girl's family had never been seriously concerned about our age differential.

At the departure gate, tears were shed by all. I naively assumed time would stand still and wait for me, but of course, this didn't happen. What did happen turned out to be not so okay, but then things will be okay for a time, until finally, way down the road, things are really not okay until I ultimately realize that not okay is really okay. Okay? Don't worry, it will become clear.

The next adventure in my life will be worth every single bit of challenge, trouble, and effort, but I won't understand the real value for almost forty years. Be assured, we are still on the path to figuring out how suicide and depression get started and then ensconced into our lives. Once we know that, we can address the roots and stop dealing with the symptoms. Speaking of symptoms, it is hard to believe that hopelessness is only a symptom, but it is. We have got to uncover the true source of hopelessness to address the fix.

What I Just Tried to Say, but in Fewer Words

- When you don't understand your root causes, all sorts of awful, unexplained, or just plain weird behavior can appear to be perfectly logical, normal, and even essential.
- All too often we think we are at fault and then pack our minds with guilt over behaviors with hidden drivers. And then to make things even worse, we take responsibility for outcomes for which we had no control.
- It is never too late to receive or give a mother's or a father's or a son's or a daughter's accepting love. The key is to give the love without attaching it to any expectation.

hy·po·der·mal

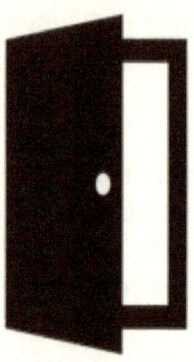

di·chot·o·my

Much earlier, I mentioned the fact that my father's acceptance of religion was the best thing that ever happened to me. This remains true, but not for any reason you might suspect. Religion, through no fault of its own, provided the perfect conduit for me to confuse success and failure into a lethal muddle that nearly ended my life.

"How," someone might ask, "can something be both lethal and the best thing that ever happened?" This is not tricky and you are probably well aware this sort of thing happens all the time. For example, water is essential for life, but too much can be deadly. Many, if not most, of our life-saving drugs, when overused, can destroy life. It is not such a stretch to see how something like religion can be misused into oblivion and that is what I came very close to doing. Apparently, I was tailor-made to take a perfectly good spirituality in a very wrong direction.

In no way do I mean to imply there is anything wrong with religion. In my particular case, I misinterpreted many aspects of religion the same way I misinterpreted many aspects of life. Each delightful misery I generated was one hundred percent my own fault, although, as you will soon

hy·po·der·mal

see, I was quite anxious to blame anybody and everybody else.

In the years since I have come to this realization, I find that now, as I look through clearer bi-focals, there were plenty of spiritual signposts that were warning me along my path, but unbeknownst to me, I was reading them upside down and backwards. I was like the dyslexic agnostic insomniac who stayed up all night wondering if there was a dog.

I volunteered for missionary service and the two years of that service brought a rich bitterness that has stretched across the ensuing decades, only to ultimately be completely replaced by a surprising sweetness. The bitterness was unexpected and supremely disappointing as I had assumed just about anything else would have resulted. The sweetness, appearing so many years later, knocked me to my knees.

I entered the prospect of missionary service with expectations of all things great and good. This was my normal starting position on most anything I undertook and as usual, I had grossly miscalculated. I pictured hours of service, helping my fellow missionaries as they helped and supported me. I could envision bringing joy and happiness to the Korean people as we shared thoughts and sought to find ways to please God together. I imagined tireless days of working with church members and neighbors in various capacities, finding great goodness in all we did. Some of this happened, but when it did, it was mostly by accident.

Don't get me wrong. I was and still am grateful for the opportunity to have served the Korean people for two years. I grew to love them and was heartbroken when I had to leave them. However, there was definitely a yin and yang thing going on. Every moment I spent with Koreans was joyful and rewarding. It was only among my fellow missionaries and mission leaders that things most often turned dark.

hy·po·der·mal

In spite of this dichotomy or maybe even because of it, there were fantastic life-altering lessons learned that I can't imagine I would have learned in any other capacity, especially at the puddin-head ages of nineteen and twenty. I entered the Land of the Morning Calm a boy and returned a man. It was a great experience, just about evenly split between joy and sorrow.

I was not and still may not be wise enough to ascertain what lie at the root of so many terrible interactions among my fellow missionaries. Some or even all may have been my own fault, but if that is the case, I was at an utter loss as to how I could have been so pervasively awful while doing everything within my power to be likeable. Just taking a statistical point of view, there were simply too many inexplicable conflicts during those two years to make sense.

My first two months were spent in a language training center to provide a foundation for learning one of the most difficult languages for an English speaker. The truth was that I didn't understand English grammar and structure all that well, so I really didn't have much of a shot at learning fluent Korean. On top of that, I had what proved to be an exceptionally low aptitude for learning a second language.

I did the very best I could, but spent the entire two months and the following two years feeling ashamed at performing far below all of my peers. This was rough on my pride, but I was determined to adopt a humble attitude and never complain. I applied this attitude with exactness when interacting with my fellow missionaries and eventually learned to laugh at myself. That lesson alone was worth all the grief.

Right from day one, we were set up in what was called companionships, in which two missionaries were made responsible to look out for each other and work together to accomplish the various tasks and duties assigned. I had imagined the two of us working to support each other and

hy·po·der·mal

becoming fast friends by virtue of our joint interests. Expectations. Expectations. Expectations.

I saw this kind of relationship develop among other sets, but my first companion never asked a single question or showed any interest in communicating with me. Instead, he managed to find a best buddy who coincidentally and instantly became my chief antagonist throughout my days in the language center and continued very enthusiastically in that same role throughout my time in Korea.

Missionaries tended to work in one part of Korea for a few months and then were routinely rotated to some different area. In a very odd and coincidental pattern, my bully preceded me in several of the areas in which I served. I was amazed to learn that I followed him time and again. It seems that as soon as he heard I was coming in to replace him, he would spread rumors among the remaining missionaries about what a terrible person I was.

At first, I had no clue he was doing this and just assumed the cold shoulders I received with each new assignment were somehow my own fault. Although it sometimes took a month or so, I was eventually able to prove to be something other than the lies that were told about me and then, much to my relief, the coldness would subside.

There were several areas in which my entire time among a group of missionaries was lonely and I felt ostracized. I remained the outsider in about half the groups with which I served. Sometimes I was able to win over some by dedication and hard work. That sort of thing was respected by just about everyone. I felt there were lots of great people in that mission, but I just didn't get to serve with many of them.

There were uncounted times I second guessed myself, wondering if I was imagining I had fallen into the center of the meanness universe. I never complained, confronted, or gave any hint of the belittlement or exclusion I experienced so often during my mission. I simply suffered in silence and

hy·po·der·mal

tried to let my efforts speak for themselves. Oh, and thank goodness for those all too rare times when someone witnessed and validated what I was experiencing. I cannot express how wonderful it was when an outsider confirmed the ill-treatment that made no sense at all to me.

About halfway through the two years, I spent five months living among a large group of missionaries. Most were fantastic people, delightful in every way, but two expressed open hatred for me from the moment we met. I have no clue why and silently endured a daily barrage of belittlements and disparaging remarks from them during our five months together. I tried to not let them affect my attitude or behavior, but I found myself doing all I could to avoid them.

On one particularly trying evening, I had received so much abuse that I had to walk outside just to clear my head. Another missionary, who happened to be serving in the capacity of an assistant to the Mission President, followed me outside and spoke with me. The Assistant said he was in awe of my ability to absorb abuse.

This was the first time anyone had ever acknowledged what I had been enduring for months. He went on to say that he would have had to shut-up anyone who spoke to him the way those two haters spoke to me. I quietly thanked him, but inside I was shouting for joy to find that I was not making up or misinterpreting all the harsh feelings that had been inexplicably directed at me.

Please understand, the vast majority of my fellow missionaries were decent types, but for whatever reason, I spent my time thrown in with the ones who seemed to enjoy picking at me. I served with both good and bad companions. Seven of the nine were actually very fine fellows and really only two qualified as difficult. One of these, during our four months together, spoke often and quite warmly with every missionary in our apartment and really every missionary we bumped into, but would go several days without speaking more than ten words to me and those were not usually very pleasant ones.

We had certain responsibilities to memorize phrases and develop a minimum ability using the native language. There were some who learned and "certified" all that was required before even leaving the language center in the States. During my two years, in spite of the fact that I spent thousands of hours studying, I never "certified," not even close. As far as I know, I am the only missionary in that mission to have failed to certify.

I left that two-year period of service filled with despair. I felt I had failed in every way I possibly could. This had nothing to do with the missionaries with whom I had served, although that didn't stop me from erroneously holding them responsible for decades. I later found my despair was a direct result of my confusion regarding the definitions of success and failure.

I had keenly observed "successful" men serving as missionaries and in other capacities throughout the church. My studies provided me with an ironclad, scripturally sound, prophetically endorsed understanding of what defines success and failure which, it turns out, could not have been more flawed if I had tried with all my might to mess it up.

I could see that all successful men and women had certain attributes and accomplishments in common and figured that if I was to be a success, I had to have those same things. I not only accrued none, not a single one, of the attributes I admired, I also had none of the accomplishments that defined my version of success.

This misunderstanding will have a mind-blowing reversal about forty years later (the great epiphany I keep referring to) and I will finally come to understand that all the decades during which I defined myself as a failure were based on a logical, but completely faulty set of premises. Stay with me, we have just a few more things to tackle before

hy·po·der·mal

we get to that point. In the meantime, I returned to my home to find things had changed. Surprise. Surprise.

What I Just Tried to Say, but in Fewer Words

- It is a **miserable** thing to link your love for someone to the expectations you have for them.
- It is a **horrific** thing to link your love for someone to completely false expectations you have for them.
- It is a **deadly thing** to link your love of yourself to completely false expectations you have for yourself.
- I heard it all my life, but never believed it. Success has little or nothing to do with outcomes (money, fame, leadership, recognition, etc.). Honestly, I used to hear this and think how completely stupid and hypocritical the person, who happened to possess all those things, sounded when spouting such drivel.
- Same goes for failure (the lack of money, fame, leadership, recognition, etc.), but only as long as you are doing about as well as you can at the time. We can make bad definitions of success and then believe with all our hearts we are failures when we are anything but that.
- Please read that previous bullet one more time. It is important.

hy·po·der·mal

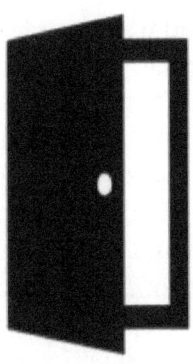

re·spite

During my first year as a missionary, I longed for the familiar, for home, for relief from the stresses and strains of learning a language and most especially, from having to deal with my fellow missionaries. During my second year, things changed, at least internally. In fact, as my term of service drew to a close, I had no desire to leave that wonderful country at all. I had fallen in love with those beautiful people.

I still spoke the worst Korean I had ever heard. I still had way too many miserable experiences with missionaries, including my companions. It turns out that by learning to love the people I served, I was the thing that had changed. It is a true tragedy that I didn't learn that same lesson for my fellow missionaries. That would have made a world of difference.

Arriving home was surreal. I was greeted at the Birmingham airport by my family and closest friends. The girl I had left behind had grown-up and was barely recognizable. I spent the night at her house and the two of us stayed up until dawn trying to figure out who the other person had become.

hy·po·der·mal

Even though we had written at least once a week to each other, I discovered she had changed in ways no letter could have revealed. I am sure the same went for me. I don't know what she thought of me, but I assumed we would simply pick up where we left off. I was wrong. The following day, she left for college in the Rocky Mountains and I enrolled in classes at home in Alabama.

It didn't take long for me to become lonely. If I was a "catch," it sure wasn't apparent from the cool reception I received for each of my social efforts. With a desperate need to connect with someone, I ended up regularly writing and phoning my now ex-girlfriend who had quickly morphed into a highly socialized and popular co-ed. She told me in great detail about all the dates she was enjoying. I continued to tele-smile, but my happy meter was flat.

Two years earlier, I had made commitments in my mind and built castles in the air on them. I was frustrated that things weren't turning out the way I assumed they would. I had not counted on a fifteen-year-old growing into an increasingly mature and independent seventeen-year-old.

Somehow, I missed the fact that with me in faraway Asia and inaccessible, I had naturally become less and less important in her own life. I was still of modest interest, but that was fading rapidly and any sort of an exclusive relationship with me was completely out of the question.

Even though I only made $2.90 per hour in my student job, I found myself calling the girl almost every day. By December, our combined phone bill had totaled $700. Tuition at that time was around $500 and we both concluded it was plainly cheaper for me to go to school out west than it was for the two of us to talk on the telephone. I applied and was accepted.

It turns out that while I was making moving plans, unbeknownst to me, the Object of My Potential Affection (OOMPA) met a handsome, wealthy, intelligent, affable, fellow named Dirt. That wasn't his actual name, but it is a

hy·po·der·mal

close approximation. As far as I could ascertain, the only problem Dirt had was a slight speech impediment from being born with a silver spoon in his mouth.

It wasn't until OOMPA came home from school for Christmas that my powers of deduction uncovered Dirt. OOMPA gave me a hint when she said, "Leave me alone. I have a handsome, wealthy, intelligent, and affable new boyfriend with a slight speech impediment. Go away. Now." Her message wasn't all that clear, so I hung around for a while.

Later that uncomfortable night, I happened to be the only one near the phone when it rang, so being polite and slightly nosey, I answered it. There was a deep, manly voice on the line asking for OOMPA. I smiled my best aw shucks grin at OOMPA and told her, "Your public is calling."

A few days later, I happened to be visiting OOMPA's family because I had asked them to invite me back and what should happen, but the phone rang again. It was midmorning and I was standing right next to it and someone asked me to answer the phone. I obliged. I was pretty sure I was talking to Dirt once again. He sounded a little surprised and asked to speak to you know who.

A little later, it occurred to me why he was surprised. OOMPA was one of four girls and except for her father, who never answered the phone, there was no brother or other male handy as a transfer operator and that begged the question, "who the dickens is this guy answering OOMPA's phone both day and night?"

About a week later, the family had me over again (this one may have been their idea). OOMPA's mood had progressed from sour to downright ugly in the meantime. It was about three in the afternoon and guess what? Ring. Ring. I was closest, so once again, I answered and whom should it be but Dirt. OOMPA seized the phone and as she walked away, I heard the dreaded words, "Oh, he's just a friend."

hy·po·der·mal

I was a "just" and that was about as much as my desperate ego was willing to take. I decided that even though I was already registered to go to school out west, I wasn't going to go. I walked out the door without saying a word to anyone, climbed into my car, and began to put this whole "dirty" situation in my rearview mirror. But then I witnessed a miracle.

OOMPA's father was a highly intelligent man who was very reserved. I had known him for several years, but had only spoken to him very few times. As I was driving away (forever as far as I was concerned), he came running out of the house and pounded on my fender.

I rolled down my window and this man who rarely spoke, pled with me to stay. He said, "Things are not always what they appear to be." He then asked me to hang around a little longer and I was so caught off guard by this remarkable occurrence that I forgot to be disgusted with OOMPA and stumbled mindlessly back into the house.

Nothing improved with OOMPA, but I decided to go out west since my tuition was only partially refundable. Driving solo in my car for two days, I arrived in the Wasatch Mountain range in the late afternoon. OOMPA had flown the same day and had been met by Dirt at the Salt Lake City airport.

Okay, things get a little crowded, so try to keep up. Oddly enough, my ex-roommate from Alabama, who knew OOMPA well, had arrived at the airport at the same time to meet his fiancé, who had just flown in from China. So now we have Dirt and OOMPA heading to the baggage area when they bump into my ex-roommate and his Chinese fiancé.

My ex-roommate says hello to OOMPA and then, before ex-roommate could say anything else, his friendly fiancé, assuming that I was the fellow holding OOMPA's hand, said hello to "me." My ex-roommate had told fiancé about me and OOMPA, so she naturally assumed I would be the fellow at the airport with OOMPA.

hy·po·der·mal

That afternoon, after my long drive, I didn't know what else to do since my wealthy socialite calendar was a blank slate, I decided to go visit OOMPA at her dormitory. I was met coolly at the door and invited inside. She left me in the hall.

Standing there in the entryway, I was invited by two of her five roommates to pitch in and move heavy stuff around the apartment. About ten minutes later, there was a knock at the door and since everyone was busy but me, I answered it. Standing there was Dirt.

It was evident I was not who or even what he had expected to answer the door. He asked for OOMPA. I pointed down the hallway and Dirt headed that direction. I didn't hear any of their conversation, but I don't think it went very well. I saw him to the door and gave him a cheery goodbye. Astonishingly, OOMPA never heard a single word from him ever again.

Sometime later, I was filled in with some facts that I had not known. It seems that Dirt had only phoned OOMPA three times over the Christmas holidays, once in the morning, once at night, and once in the afternoon, spread over a ten-day period. I had answered every one of his calls and apparently that had given him the impression I lived there.

He then went to the airport and was accosted and mistaken as me by two complete strangers, one of them an international traveler. He came by to visit OOMPA and had been cheerfully greeted at the door by yours truly. You can see he was getting a rather skewed picture of reality by this time and from his perspective, I appeared to be an omnipresent, unstoppable force.

Suffice to say that through a very peculiar set of coincidences, the new boyfriend lost interest and I ended up marrying my ex-girlfriend the last day of spring that same year. She was eighteen and I was twenty-one and for the first time in my life, I felt secure in a relationship, although there were other factors and influences still in flux. Finally, I felt accepted.

Over the next five years, I graduated with a couple of degrees and during this emotional oasis, I managed to develop some lasting friendships and one in particular, inspired me to improve some aspects of my character. A fellow, who was a second-year law student, had the ability to merge and intertwine the logic of the world with the logic of religion in such a way that it shook me to the core.

Even though I had served as a full-time missionary, most of what I had done had been based on a combination of shallow understanding, sheer determination, and deep faith. Now I had a chance to start deepening my weak understanding. I became much more sincere in all my studies, ultimately developing a tremendous thirst for knowledge in numerous fields. Shockingly, my grades improved. Who would have thought studying helped?

I was twenty-seven years old and finally feeling pretty good about who I had become for the first time in my life. I had a wife who loved me unquestioningly and I had proved the mettle to graduate from college with better than average grades. On top of that, I had developed some lasting friendships with people who stuck by me through thick and thin. This was the longest period of my life in which I could say I was happy.

I took my first professional job in southern California, hired by a man for unclear reasons that were never explained to me. He was a powerful director of a large aircraft company and I had been brought in as his assistant. I sat in an office across from his for nine months without one single meaningful assignment. During the entire time, I had maybe five total hours of anything work-related to do. I asked, offered, begged, and pled for work, but all to no avail.

Every now and then I was given some small organizational task that might take an hour to complete, but for the most part I was bored and desperate for something to

hy·po·der·mal

fill the long, unbearable hours. At the end of those nine miserable months, I was transferred into a highly sought after fast-track career program filled with super-smart people with whom I had no business competing. Through a bizarre twist of fate, I ended up in another position in which I basically spent fifteen months doing a whole bunch of nothing while watching my cohorts launch incredible careers.

Being paid to do nothing was morally contrary to everything I believed. I wanted to work, I just wasn't allowed to. I only complained a single time and it happened to be to the vice-president of Marketing. We had met and he saw I was willing to work and thought I might fit in very well with his team.

Getting out of my fast-track program was going to be a little tricky. My potential new boss spoke with the president of the company, who then spoke with the director who had hired me and then moved heaven and earth to get me instated in the fast-track program. The director did not appreciate my attitude and told me if I ever did anything like that to embarrass him again, he would crucify me. I believed him and immediately started looking for a new job.

Just before the beginning of our third year in SoCal, we had our first child and decided to leave my do-nothing rat race and try our hand at starting our own business. We took all the money we had saved to buy a house and purchased the goods to open a retail craft store in Salt Lake City, Utah. I had zero interest in everything we sold, but we timed our entry right and managed to corner the market for a few years with our business growing 300% per year for four years in a row. We grossed a million dollars in our fourth year.

Starting a new business is expensive and difficult, but I helped to make ends meet the first year by hiring on with a large company at which I was paid to do nothing for the entire time I stayed there. I never took a job expecting to do nothing. I always assumed I was hired and paid for doing

hy·po·der·mal

something. Sadly, this same thing will happen many times in the coming years. Some might want these circumstances, I didn't.

Once our business was self-sustaining, I quit my third do-nothing job. I had now spent three years in the professional world and had received lots of paychecks but no practical experience. I really tried, but I couldn't bring myself to enjoy selling the frilly fopdoodles we stocked, so I mostly occupied my time with constructing store expansions and the overhead functions of running a going enterprise. We enjoyed six major expansions, growing from 600 square feet to over 13,000 in three years.

I was happiest when I had a building project or when spending time with my daughter and wife. In fact, even though this period in my life was difficult and stressful in many ways, the problems were all external and easily handled. I had a stable relationship, some friends, a daughter, and soon we added a son. My internal workings were humming and I felt better than I ever had before.

I began to believe I had overcome my shortcomings, my triggers, and my feelings of inadequacy. I assumed because I was maturing, I had become wiser and that was the source of my positive outlook. I had no idea I was sitting on a fault-line that only needed a good shake to resurrect my old miseries.

Just as with any married couple, we had our disagreements, but for seven years, not a single one of our disputes had been personal. We had learned the give and take that all committed couples must learn in order to grow closer. One afternoon in December of 1987, for the first time in our marriage, things got personal and even though I did everything within my power to let it go, I didn't have the ability. I was still carrying my same old triggers, I just didn't know it.

We were discussing the imbalance of demands on our time or some such matter and at one point the subject turned

hy·po·der·mal

to how I was using my own time. I felt a little insecure because not only did I genuinely detest selling ribbons and lace, but I had never done any real professional work and unless I was building something for our store, I often felt lazy and useless. I wanted to do more to help, but there was something in me that was repulsed by the very business that was providing so well for us. I suppose I felt it was superficial.

My wife, for some long forgotten reason, turned what I thought was a perfectly normal discussion into a direction we had never ventured before. She began to question what I was doing with regard to church service. I felt I was pretty dedicated and was meeting my obligations for the most part, but then she said something that I never expected to come from her lips. Once again, I had developed a faulty expectation and linked my emotions to it.

She had gotten a little heated and claimed I was a hypocrite, talking a good talk, but not actually doing any of the work I claimed I was doing. It is possible that some aspect of what she was saying was correct at a given moment, but I had never expected my trusted partner to disparage me, especially in an area where I had always felt I had consistently done my best. I had an expectation that she would never attack my character and when that happened, something inside me cracked.

I felt innocent and betrayed, but to my credit, I simply collapsed physically and mentally. My triggers, as often as they had gotten me into hot water, were a little rusty and I was dedicated to treating my wife as gentlemanly as I was capable. I had established an unbreakable code in that regard. Slumping into a chair, I sat there for several hours, unmoving, so emotionally distraught that I began physically hurting.

As the sun set, I felt a sensation that is unique in my life. I am not sure how to describe it, but to say there was a splitting inside my head. It felt as though an opening in my mind appeared and something dark and evil crept inside. I sank into an ever deepening depression over the next months and never felt the same about my wife. I had lost a small measure of trust in her and could no longer be completely certain she was looking out for my best interest. We had enjoyed seven wonderful years, but this was the beginning of something not good.

Looking in from the outside, it is very easy to examine this situation and sincerely ask, "What's the big deal?" I was a person of undying, unwavering loyalty, but I also had the terrible attribute of ascribing my own characteristics as normal and setting equal expectations on others. Of course, I didn't have the same level of expectation for all attributes and I understood that people have different abilities and talents as well as shortcomings and flaws. But with my background and experiences, there were a couple of things that were for all intents and purposes, untouchable. Protection and trust of a spouse was one of those – and it went both ways.

I had known without a shadow of a doubt my wife had my best interests at heart and would never knowingly try to undermine or hurt me, even in anger. Once she violated that trust, I began to revert into my old thinking patterns. I probably had no clue what was happening, but that didn't stop it from continuing on into the darkness. I just knew I had lost something precious and try as I might, I couldn't seem to get it back.

Other than my depression, I never gave a clue to my wife what I was feeling, mostly because I couldn't have put it into words. And I won't be able to for at least another twenty years, but the crack was now there and my respite was starting to crumble.

My wife became convinced I had clinical depression. I went to a specialist and not surprisingly, I was indeed diagnosed with clinical depression. "Sir, take these pills.

hy·po·der·mal

Please leave a big bag of money with our receptionist on your way out, thank you very much."

At the time, I blindly accepted this diagnosis, although there was a nagging voice inside me that said something else was at the root of my distraught emotions. The quack who prescribed the drugs for me gave me four times the normal dosage of an ancient psychotropic drug that had rarely been used for years due to its terrible side-effects. I enjoyed each and every one in a colorful horror-kaleidoscope and almost lost my mind.

After two years of feeling like I was imprisoned inside my own head, I quit cold turkey and life soon resumed to some version of normal. I wondered about this concept of depression, thinking to myself what if the real cause is something other than an imbalance of chemicals? What if I was feeling whatever it was I was feeling because I was supposed to feel that way given my understanding and interpretation of my circumstances? I was dead spot on, but didn't know it.

I had defined my life such that I could only fail and had no clue I had done so. I thought I was doing things correctly and suspected that everything about which I felt so despondent were things that would be normal to feel despondent about. This was not exactly the case, but it was definitely part of the picture. Little did I know that it was my thinking, not my chemicals, which was causing me to sink deeper and deeper into depression. Intuitively, I knew this to be true, but it would take another twenty years to completely expose this truth to the light.

Please don't mistake my meaning to imply there is no such thing as chemical depression. It is real. What I am saying is that it might be a part of the root cause or maybe not. It is possible to have "stinkin' thinkin'" and still have other medical issues. However, it is also possible that anti-depressants are providing a chemical mask, hiding the underlying root of a problem.

hy·po·der·mal

I know, at least in my own case, it is possible to treat symptoms without ever treating the cause. As you will soon learn, I had one of the worst cases of stinkin' thinkin' in history (possibly a slight exaggeration) and even if I had chemical depression, it was essential that I find what was poisoning me besides a lack of serotonin. The good news is I did.

What I Just Tried to Say, but in Fewer Words

- Happiness and emotional stability are rarely related and stability is the one that counts. Having a mind at peace allows happiness and sadness to play equally important and equally desirable roles. I know, I know, that sounds like pure pony poop and if I hadn't lived it for over three years so far, while standing knee deep in said pony poop, I would be laughing at me right along with you.
- Until you address root causes, you are only dealing with symptoms.
- The saddest and by far most deadly aspect of only addressing symptoms is when we think we are backsliding. We are not backsliding at all. The roots are still in play.

hy·po·der·mal

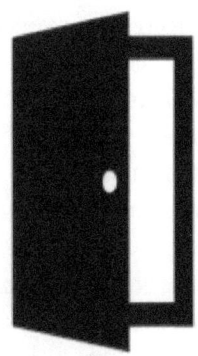

os·cil·la·tion

I thought I had led a schizophrenic life in the mission field with joy and misery swinging back and forth like a windy gate and constantly warring for my attention, but the period I am about to enter is a mood typhoon. I now knew it was possible for my wife to willingly hurt me, but that didn't mean she would ever do it again. I put all my energy into positive thoughts and avoided anything that might damage our relationship.

My wife was carrying a heavy load with our growing family and a business that would suck every second of life from her if it could. She really performed remarkably well under such pressure, much better than I ever could. There were a few things she felt negatively about me and gradually began to share these concerns more and more often. I began to dread our "discussion" time.

I desperately wanted and needed to be accepted for what I was in the moment, not for what I used to be and not for what I might one day become. I didn't have a clue that was what I needed at the time, but it was true, nevertheless. I began to hear words that were probably well intended, but given my background, I was forced to translate them as "you are not good enough."

hy·po·der·mal

I was specifically told on several occasions, "You are not the man I married." I couldn't comprehend it at the time, but these words were slamming directly into the heart of my hidden four-year-old and my already fractured trust began to seriously erode under the onslaught.

After repeated and increasing hammerings, all sorts of conflicts sprouted and grew up as weeds in my mind, haunting me. Try as I might, I couldn't help but have some of my frustrations spill out into the world, sometimes at perfect strangers and sometimes at loved ones. As that kind of behavior increased, I began to lose hope that I would ever be acceptable to anyone.

The more I did what I hated, the more I hated myself and then the more I would do what I hated. You see where that was headed. I began to contemplate my own death. It took a while, but eventually I learned to keep the majority of this darkness to myself. I grew to no longer trust my wife with my innermost thoughts, fearing that exposing my soul would only net me more abuse.

Sadly, there were a few times I shared my worries with her and they came back to hurt me in the form of compounded criticisms. It truly is a greater thing to be trusted than loved. Love is easy. Trust, once lost, is very difficult to restore. I still loved, but I no longer trusted, at least not with the things of my heart.

Let me make something perfectly clear. I am not accusing my wife of doing any of this vindictively. It is my opinion she thought she was doing what needed to be done and had no idea of the destruction that was happening inside me. I could feel it, but I couldn't understand it, much less explain it.

She had never had to work or live under the dismal circumstances and abuse that I did. She couldn't comprehend the triggers and scars that were involved regardless of her good or bad intentions. My wife had plenty on her own plate and much like a drowning person, she was grasping for whatever would save her own life under the circumstances.

Unfortunately, the reasons for her actions made no difference at all regarding the trust that I was gradually losing. I really only had one need and although it took several long years before I could put it into words, I eventually discovered it was essential that my wife somehow accept me with all my faults. That didn't mean she had to approve of them or not try to help me overcome them. I just needed someone to say I was worth keeping, even if I never got any better.

It didn't matter that she may have had a good or innocent reason to not accept the current version of me. Rejection was betrayal as far as I was concerned, even for a good reason. Betrayal was a trigger with roots too deep to overcome without skills far beyond what I possessed at that time.

I knew it was possible to accept someone with all their faults because I accepted my wife no matter what she did. Even when betraying me, I tried to not hold it against her and focused on all her great qualities. I genuinely admired her, giving her all I had to give. I almost succeeded in holding on to my deep love for her in spite of the fact that I no longer trusted her, but then she started involving my children in the betrayal process and that was more than I could overcome. I will address this nightmare later.

As I felt the holes grow inside me, I began searching for fulfilment once more. I understood that I was committed in marriage and would have never, ever stepped outside of any boundaries, but I did gain an understanding of why some spouses do. In fact, I wouldn't even get close to an edge, but I recognized that something essential in my life was missing. I hadn't yet developed the insight to understand exactly what, but I was learning what it wasn't. Another ten years will pass before I clearly understood my desperate need to be accepted for who I was. Not surprisingly, this was the

hy·po·der·mal

exact same thing I needed from my mother and in some ways, every other woman.

Like many who feel undefined needs, I mostly looked outside of myself for answers. I decided to learn to play the guitar. This seemed like a useful skill and it was one I had always felt would be worthwhile. Over a five or six year period, I went through about a dozen expensive guitars, buying high and selling low. I lost thousands of dollars. Each purchase felt right until I brought it home, then something would feel wrong. I learned to play "Can't Buy Me Love," but I didn't understand the obvious message.

If you are looking for trouble identifiers, this behavior would have stood out very brightly from the crowd. Looking back, I can now see it was obvious that something was amiss. I was trying to fill a void. I used guitars. Some people use shoes, clothes, jewelry, sports, guns, or most terrifyingly, other people to meet an internal yearning. We all, sooner or later, discover an external answer never satisfies an internal question.

In desperation, I thought I could find happiness in a purposeful career. I looked into medical school, architectural school, and starting a computer repair business. As I attempted each of these paths, something insurmountable would appear and I would move on to the next idea. In 1990, I was asked to teach religious classes at a local high school in an unpaid position. I did this for a year and a half and even though it was very time consuming and demanding, I enjoyed interacting with the kids.

I liked teaching enough to try to use it as a means to fill my void. I had no clue it would have never done so, but I was willing to try. After being urged to apply for a paid position for the coming year, I interviewed and seemed to be well thought of, but after all was said and done, I was told I was not "orthodox" enough to be accepted into the program. I had no idea what that meant, but I had received a premonition that just such a thing would happen and managed to accept that particular rejection without any external fuss. Internally, I was a mess.

Once I no longer had my daily teaching commitment, I searched for some other way to make a positive impact in the world. I decided to volunteer to serve in one of my church's organizations two days a week. Again, much like the teaching position, it was demanding, but very rewarding. After about a year and a half, it dawned on me what I was really doing was hiding from my responsibilities and I was still trying to fill that missing component in my life.

Our business had done very well for a while, but severe competition had muscled in next door and soon we began to flounder. I stopped my volunteer work and sought some way to help make ends meet. For about three months, I was hired into a temporary position to design a marketing catalogue for a local business. I was well paid, but more importantly, I was appreciated. It had been a long time since I had felt appreciated in any sort of professional or private sense. This provided a feeling of satisfaction I hadn't experienced for several years.

During all this time of steady depression with short breaks, the only aspect in my life in which I believed I was succeeding was fatherhood. I spent countless hours reading to my children every night of their lives. I was the one who put our children to bed, bathed them, and rocked them to sleep. I read hundreds of books by nightlight, sitting on the floor as they dozed off one by one. Even though I have very little talent for it, I sang for hours at a time as I rocked and held each of my little ones in my arms. In my mind, I understood I was not perfect, but I truly felt I was doing the very best I was capable of doing.

This is an important observation because in the coming years I will be told many times how I have fallen short as a father, mostly from my wife, but also from my children. I will react very badly sometimes when this happens and considering my triggers regarding abused innocence and

hy·po·der·mal

betrayal, it will be a miracle that I didn't react any more badly than I did.

There will come a day when my wife will admit that she purposefully undermined my relationships with my children and she will have done this because she believed with all her heart it was the right thing to do. She was not a bad person or mother, but she had her own version of stinkin' thinkin'. I suspect we all do to lesser and greater degrees.

Her undermining will be the event of betrayal that finally obliterates my ability to accept my wife no matter what she does. I will continue to love her and admire her qualities, but even my incredible loyalty and level of deep commitment have their limits. There is a very dark time ahead, but we need to look at some of the interim stuff before we enter that world.

In 1997, our business collapsed and I was forced to return to the full-time working world with my three years of nothing experience and ten years of owning a business in which I did very little. My resume stunk, but I needed a big salary for my growing family. We moved back to Alabama and even though job opportunities were practically non-existent, I was hired for a temporary position in a sawmill as an engineer. Astonishingly, I was once more given absolutely nothing to do.

This time I was determined to find something meaningful to fill my fifty hour work-week and try the best I could to deserve my paycheck. I searched for needs, invented every one of my assignments, and surprisingly seemed to produce something worthwhile after everything was said and done. This was one of the few times I ever productively earned my salary.

After the contract ended, it was three long months before I found another job. During that hiatus, I shattered my right leg, twisting it such that only my skin held the pieces together. The uselessness I felt at being a father of six, unable to walk, and unemployed plunged me to an all-

hy·po·der·mal

time low. I spent months in bed and was in real danger of giving up, but for a couple of unexpected and inspiring events.

One day, I woke up and a stranger was mowing my lawn. It turned out he was a man who I didn't really know very well and how he knew we needed his help was never explained. As soon as he was done, he left without saying a word. On another day, the elderly woman living next door came into my bedroom and carefully handed me a hundred dollar bill. She told me that God had instructed her to do it. Little acts of kindness and my own loving children kept me afloat during this tragedy. Unfortunately, I will set several new record lows during the next five years.

In my next employment opportunity, I was hired just as I was learning to walk using crutches. Once again, I had nothing to do. I struggled, searching for some way to contribute and eventually invented a revenue source for the company by developing storm-water control presentations for government entities.

My boss was one of the most horrible and cartoonish characters I ever knew. After just one year, I fled to what would be the one and only job I ever held that was meaningful right from the start. I was given an amazing partner and together with a big bag of federal money, we zoomed around the state of Alabama for a year providing all sorts of services and aids for small mom and pop manufacturers.

Unfortunately, the corrupt man in charge of our efforts had the skill to pin his wrong-doing on me and before he could crush me under his greed, I managed to flee to another job in which I had nothing to do, but this time I was separated by 200 miles from my family. I spent a miserable year in south Alabama, only returning to my little ones on the weekends, but it was better than saying to the camera on the courthouse steps, "Yes, that is my signature, but no, that is not my yacht."

hy·po·der·mal

The depression during this time was palatable. I was still faithfully providing for my wife and children, but the dread of each long, lonely, useless week caused me to sink into a deep darkness which try as I might, I could not shake off during the weekends with my family.

It was at this low point my wife said something that I believed to be true at the time, but it wasn't even close to true. I know she didn't mean her words to impact me the way they did, but what she said affected me as badly as being told my mother hated me or at least it was a very close second.

She was doing the best she could while juggling seven children with the eighth on the way and frankly, was really performing incredibly by anyone's standard. I was not very helpful in my depressed state and in her frustration she lashed out at me. She was disgusted that I was so depressed on weekends. I could understand why she felt that way with her life being packed to the gills as it was.

The problem was that I was barely functioning at all. The dread of being away from my family and having to go to a place where I was forced to appear busy even though I had nothing to do while working among a hostile bunch of co-workers was destroying me. The hostility had started when my boss placed me on probation for not appreciating my co-worker's criticisms properly. I had been severely and publicly chastened for speaking to another co-worker about a negative part of our responsibilities and was told by my chastener that I had engaged in inappropriate behavior.

I was forty-two years old and figured I had a pretty good idea of what was appropriate and what behavior to avoid, so I politely, but firmly refuted his accusation by saying I had not done anything wrong. He immediately ran to our boss, his best friend, and suddenly I was enemy number one. This was something straight out of junior high school and made an already unbearable situation much worse.

hy·po·der·mal

One weekend, as my spouse was really struggling under a particularly busy load, she told me she was no longer happy with me and that she didn't think she deserved such a husband. She said she couldn't bear the thought of having a depressed man like her father had been. Then she said something that was devastating on many levels. She told me that for the past twenty years, she had been carrying the entire load of our family solely upon her own shoulders. This was rough to hear.

Then she added that she had long ago decided to wall off all emotions for me rather than feel constant anger for my shortcomings. Even though I knew she hadn't had loving feelings for me for years, it was still hard to hear. The combination of her two statements would have been devastating even if I hadn't been in such deep darkness for so long.

I believed every word she said, especially the part of how she had been carrying the family by herself. My feelings of failure fit like hand in glove to that sentiment. I would suffer unnecessarily for years before I realized she was completely wrong.

As you might imagine, I sank to an all-time low believing I had failed in every aspect of my life. I had spent my career doing nothing while having to pretend I was busy and was currently hated by my coworkers and boss in a job two hundred miles away. I had failed as a missionary in every conceivable way, having never served in any meaningful capacity and I hadn't even been able to learn the language. I had never been asked to serve in any noteworthy way in my church or community. The only job I ever enjoyed had been ruined by a greedy manager and I had to leave because I could see I was being set up to take the fall for some wrongdoing.

Every other woman in my life had abandoned me and now there was one more. My wife thought I was a failure and told me my children were constantly disappointed with

hy·po·der·mal

me. As a husband, I was decimated when she said out loud that she had to consciously stop feeling any emotions just to be able to tolerate me and not outright hate me. I was once again that little boy who felt betrayed by the one woman who he never expected to betray him.

Amazingly, I kept going in spite of all this drag. I wanted to shut down, but I never stopped. I dreaded every moment of my life except when I was with my children. I spent hours sitting in the silent dark, listening to the voices in my head scream at me to just kill myself, but I fought against them with the tiny bit of life still left inside me. In retrospect, it is quite a success that I refused to let the depression prevent me from providing for my family.

Because I believed all that my wife had said, I lost all hope. This is a very dangerous condition for anyone. Once there is no hope, a vacuum develops which is soon filled with the darkest of thoughts. Nothing is good enough. Nothing matters. I didn't realize it then, but that was possibly the strongest and greatest moment of my life. I couldn't have known it at the time and I certainly wouldn't have believed it, but the very moment I felt I was the greatest failure, I was actually living one of my greatest successes: Not giving up was a tremendous victory.

For months, I felt nothing and no longer could even understand why I needed to keep breathing. Yet, somehow I managed to keep going to that terrible job, living alone in a miserable tiny cinderblock apartment. Every day I spent all day hiding and disguising my non-work from the prying eyes of my adversarial co-workers trying to get me fired. All the while, I was being told by my wife I was not what she wanted nor what she had signed up for as she walled off her emotions in order to avoid actively hating me. Day after horrible day, I kept battling for an entire year.

I was desperate to find another job and was finally offered a position in a Mississippi sawmill making caskets, coincidentally also 200 miles away from my family. My

hy·po·der·mal

first day of work, a co-worker got angry with me and swung a board at my head. My boss, who proved to be the second most horrible boss in my life, told me it was my fault and to shut up and quit whining. Everything went downhill after that with the exception of one thing, this time I had my oldest son and daughter living with me while the rest of my family stayed in Alabama awaiting the birth of child number eight. Those two were my salvation.

The job proved to be a nightmare in every conceivable way. I had interviewed for one position, but ended up being placed into an entirely different one for which I had no qualifications. This was a brand new position, not even defined yet, and once again I had absolutely nothing to do.

I struggled to find some way to fill my hours, usefully if possible, but it was very difficult. I often wondered at the amazing track record I had of taking jobs with nothing to do over and over, it was much stranger than fiction. Why did I keep getting hired at all? There was nothing on my resume that didn't look downright spooky. I had no real experience at anything and I changed jobs every year. If I was an employer, I wouldn't have touched me with a ten-foot pole.

After the birth of number eight, the whole family moved to Mississippi and it was not a good fit for anyone as everyone struggled with the change. My job was spiraling out of control with my boss trying to force me into doing something unethical and probably illegal. I had also accidentally overheard our corporate leaders were trying to close our facility. I began searching for my sixth job in as many years and landed one in Missouri in 2002. This time I was so far away from my family that I only saw them one weekend in a two month period until they joined me.

Fortunately, I had finally found a job in which I was appreciated. Not surprisingly, I had nothing to do, but this time there were things needed in this business I could actually provide. I only worked there two years, but during that time my boss was named employee of the world for the

hy·po·der·mal

company and I had a little bit to do with him receiving that honor.

Part of my family thrived in Missouri and part fell apart. Once again, there was some corporate rumblings that our facility might be on the chopping block, so I decided for the sake of my family's security, I needed to start searching for my seventh job in eight years. I hated leaving a job for which I was considered a major asset. When I turned in my notice, my boss teared up. That was a first.

In 2004, we moved to Huntsville, Alabama and I took employment in which I had, you guessed it, nothing to do. I was hired as a consultant to find cost savings in the United States Army. This sounded fantastic, but the problem was that actual cost savings resulted in managers being punished for making inaccurate budgets.

If managers spent exactly what was in their budget, they were rewarded with bigger budgets. If not, they were publicly castigated for being terrible and stupid budgeters. Then they would have their budgets cut so that "smart" budgeters could spend bigger budgets. Guess how many were interested in saving money in their budget? I was forced to look extremely busy while doing absolutely nothing.

It is amazing how creatively nothing can be described as a whole bunch of something. Using the term "Cost Avoidance" instead of "Cost Savings" was the key. Imagine that a toilet seat normally costs $15,000 and you find one for only $7,000. Why you just provided the U.S. Government a cost avoidance of $8,000! You can see if you buy enough $7,000 toilet seats, you can quickly cost avoidance into some real money. Just imagine not buying $20,000 toilet seats! Don't slip on the dripping sarcasm.

After one year of this madness, I realized that I was basically stealing the taxpayer's money and I found that to be morally reprehensible. Job number eight in nine years appeared when I converted to a government position in

hy·po·der·mal

which I was asked to do nothing for three years. I switched to another position during which I have now been heavily involved in "cost avoidance" for ten years. Wink. Wink.

I share this employment history and the accompanying insights with the hope that you will see there was rarely anything worthwhile happening outside my own family. I felt forced to stake my self-worth on my familial relationships. Everything else was a catastrophe.

I had very few friends, basically no hobbies, and nearly every one of my jobs had not only been worthless, but some were despicable. The only thing that kept me sane regarding my employment was that if I didn't have whatever position I had, someone else would have it and at least I was using the money to raise a beautiful family.

As you can see, there were both bad and good things happening during this oscillating period, but everything was always creeping steadily downward, particularly regarding the thing that mattered most to me, my family.

We are just about done with roots and everything that lies ahead has all the appearance of failure and it many ways it actually is failure. But much like that dark, dark period in which I continued to plod along with no hope, sometimes actual failure is anything but what it appears to be. A little more darkness and then we finally hit the light.

What I Just Tried to Say, but in Fewer Words

- Kindness can save lives. You can stop a death spiral in yourself or others by performing a simple act of kindness or service. It doesn't always work on the first try, but if you make several sincere attempts, something magical happens and perspectives always, I repeat, always change. Always. This sounds so stupid it has to be true and it is.

hy·po·der·mal

- Accepting someone with their faults does not mean you accept their faults and frankly, a person is really dumb if they don't understand this.

P.S. During this period of my life I met a man who was impressive. His new born daughter had been erroneously given a drug that was specifically prohibited on her medical chart. The result was that his first born child would spend the rest of her life severely challenged. I grew to love that little girl and one day I asked her father how he maintained such an incredible peace given all the difficulties in his life. He told me he had learned two things, "First, don't sweat the small stuff and second, everything is small stuff." I thought that was witty and pretty smart, but I didn't understand the deeper meaning at the time. I do now and if you don't already, you will too in just a bit.

hy·po·der·mal

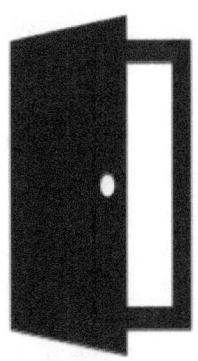

sab·o·tage

In spite of the fact that I was convinced I had failed in just about everything that mattered in life, I somehow maintained enough will to get out of bed every day and fulfil my responsibilities. There were days when I was right on the edge of giving up, but then I would realize that there really was no excuse for such cowardice. I hated cowards, always have. I had some wonderful children who were still young enough to not realize what a total failure their father was and that gave me some moments of peace, but still I wondered if they would not be better off without me.

Other than being with my kids, my best moments occurred when I was in the process of accomplishing something I could both touch and see. Combining kids and building projects was nirvana. If I was building some structure or remodeling a section of our house, the progress of each day could create such happiness in me that the world seemed perfectly right and worth living in.

During these times I slept like the dead and bounced out of bed, impatient to get started on whatever was next. There was a particularly wonderful period between 2005 and 2008 in which I built a three-car garage, a movie room with built-in crows nests complete with a hammock for little guys to

hy·po·der·mal

get a bird's eye view, and a four-story, 500 square-foot castle with drawbridge, curly slide, climbing wall, and two massive towers (with trap doors) connected by a twenty-foot high bridge. Oh, and a twelve-foot fireman's pole, too.

This pleasant period just preceded my turning fifty-years of age. With the single exception of my spectacular broken leg eleven years earlier, my health had always been outstanding. I was very active and my weight had not varied much since I was in my twenties. However some sort of genetic switch activated in 2008. A friend noticed that I was breathing hard while we were walking and said he thought that was something to look into. I had just hoofed it up a hill and really thought he was being silly.

A few weeks later, I went in for my annual physical and my doctor decided he wanted to check out my heart. This was something new and I figured it was just part of the routine of getting older. After the EKG, he said he found a little something and we argued for ten minutes that he was only trying to run up his bill so he could build more money forts. We were old friends and he finally guilted me into seeing a specialist. Two stents later in the artery my heart surgeon called "the widow maker," I was given a new lease on life.

I took my new lease and promptly developed sleep apnea, diabetes, bad eyesight, deafness, high blood pressure, gastric reflux, stomach polyps, a ruptured and replaced C-7 disc, tinnitus, a hiatal hernia, punctured lungs and broken ribs, high cholesterol, all flavors of bad triglycerides, and most delightfully, hemorrhoids. Oh yeah, and nine, count them, nine kidney stones. I went from zero prescriptions to owning a private pharmacy in three short years. Throughout these health disturbances, I refused to give up working outside and doggedly pursued the kinds of projects that filled me with joy.

Then one day in 2011, I thought something had gone wrong with my hips. I went to see a half dozen specialists,

hy·po·der·mal

each telling me that I had no arthritis and my hips were fine. Apparently they were right, but still I was barely able to walk and in 2014, I sought out a highly recommended British neurosurgeon teaching and practicing at one of the nearby medical schools. He agreed with his fellow practitioners, saying my hips were fine, but he did wonder that none of them had noticed the inch-long crack in my spine.

It turns out that I had been living with a broken back, a fractured L-5 vertebrae, for three years at that point. My doctor said that there was no explanation for why it wouldn't heal and he made sure of this by charging me for two of every test he could think of. His money fort added a guest house.

After running out of options, he recommended that I live with the pain for as long as I could and only opt for surgery when I could no longer function. I promptly celebrated by gaining seventy-five pounds and giving up all the activities that had kept me sane.

Now, with the completion of this medical history, we are ready to proceed into my darkest days with a pretty good understanding of just about all of the pre-contributors to my upcoming depression. Along with my terrible job and failing marriage, I was riddled with pain, but somehow kept going into work every day. Walking was nearly impossible and by the end of each day, I was shot.

During this time, several of my children had achieved adulthood or would shortly be reaching that stage. It was at this point I felt most vulnerable regarding the manly things which I was no longer able to perform and unfortunately, my wife picked this time to significantly accelerate and express her dissatisfaction with her husband. Her timing could not have been more devastating.

Complaints started to accrue and regular sessions were scheduled to change me. It seems I wasn't attending enough choir concerts or sporting events. I was told my children were saying these things, but I never heard them myself. I suspected my children weren't actually saying these things at all, but it was my wife interpreting, inferring, and possibly even manufacturing such attitudes. I was instructed that I didn't listen properly and had failed to seek out opportunities to visit with each child to hear his or her concerns, complaints, and accomplishments.

This was rough on me because I believed I was doing the absolute best I could do under the circumstances and frankly, I thought I was doing an excellent job in spite of my difficulties. Whenever I had even a tiny chance to interface with my kids, I seized it with great enthusiasm – especially in the rare event that they had sought me out. I still cared greatly for my wife, but she had become increasingly distant and cold and it wasn't long until we grew mostly silent with one another.

Time for an important reminder: Please understand this is my story, told with my prejudices and my point of view. I believe I am telling the whole truth and nothing but the truth, but that doesn't mean it is the only truth. Other's truths are just as important and may conflict with my own. Nonetheless, I can only present this story as I believe it to be. I have no desire to paint my wife or anyone else in a false light. These are the facts as I understand them.

My children were the only things that brought me any kind of joy at this time of my life and I did everything within my power to build up relationships with them. Being constantly told I had failed and was destined to continue failing with them was devastating because I knew I was giving my all. I had not yet learned to suspect my wife, so each accusation added to my accumulating failures and to my darkness.

I believed everything my wife told me until one day it occurred to me that she may have an ulterior motive. I had never thought anything but that she had the best of intentions. I knew she was not perfect, but I was nothing, if

hy·po·der·mal

not loyal and defended her good name even between my own ears.

This new thought came after pondering for months how I could be such a terrible father after doing all within my power to be the best I knew how to be. I was aware that maybe my best was not very good, but I was tender, attentive, extremely mild, a creative and gentle disciplinarian, and when asked for any attention, I always responded.

The first time I had felt any suspicion was when she told me my son wanted a closer relationship, although he had never said a word to me about it and we seemed to have a wonderful time whenever we were together. Besides, what good son or daughter wouldn't want a better relationship with a parent?

At first, I focused on my son and gradually came to realize that he may indeed have some of those feelings, but rather than encouraging my son to talk with me, my wife had chosen to speak directly to me about my shortcomings. I didn't find out until later that had been a long standing pattern of hers.

I realized a desire for more attention from my son was not actually a problem, it was the norm when it came to teens. I suspected a mild form of betrayal was occurring right under my nose, probably with the best of intentions, but my spouse was instigating problems rather than helping. I reacted with frustration, not yet understanding the real root of my thinking.

Once I realized that sabotage was a possibility, I began to increase my awareness of not just what was being said to me, but how and when it was being reported. I immediately noted that whatever complaint I was facing, it was always from my wife and never from my children. I began to question her reports, seeking out my children to see if they agreed. Sometimes they did and sometimes they were as surprised as I was.

hy·po·der·mal

My wife may have done this because she believed in the righteousness of her cause regarding our children, but I gradually came to see how detrimental this kind of divisiveness can be to a marriage. It didn't take me long to learn an absolute, irrefutable truth regarding marriage. You can marry your spouse or you can marry something else, such as your children or your job, but you can't marry both and honestly hope for a healthy relationship. If your spouse isn't your top priority most of the time, the marriage may very well survive, but it will never thrive. Don't ever let anyone tell you this isn't true. It is.

Like so many married couples, we began having the exact same discussion over and over. Of course, I can't begin to express what was going on in my wife's mind, but I can present my own thoughts. Some issue would arise and we would begin a sincere exploration of what can be done. Inevitably, the conversation would turn to something along the lines of "we need to improve." I would agree and quickly and willingly name specific things I had been doing poorly and what I could do about them. I would then ask my wife, the other half of "we," what she might do to improve.

The same thing happened more times than I can count. She would respond by asking me what I thought she should do. I would respond by saying I didn't have any complaints and I didn't want her to change a thing, I just "needed to be needed." She would ask for clarification and I would stumble along the best I could, but never could give her an answer she seemed to understand.

I now realize I was asking to be accepted for who I was at that moment with the trust that I would improve over time, BUT IF I NEVER CHANGED, I was still a great guy and perfectly acceptable as is. It wasn't that I didn't plan on changing for the better, I absolutely did, I just needed to know that even if I didn't, I was good enough.

These repetitive discussions always ended in the exact same fashion with both of us frustrated and me saying,

hy·po·der·mal

"Please stop trying to change me. I am a good person just the way I am." She would always reply, "You know you must change, we all have to change." I would then attempt to explain I was not talking about specific behaviors, but about my character itself and round and round we went.

I knew I had lived a very good life, with relatively few experiences in which I had known to do right and chosen to do wrong. I had committed tens of thousands of bad choices in the heat of the moment, but for the most part, when given sufficient time to consider, I chose well. Our discussion conclusion was always a plea from my wife for counseling in which "we" would get help. We went to multiple counselors and it didn't take long for me to figure out "we" meant "me."

The two of us must have found and met multiple times with three of the most idiotic therapists in the world. Even my wife agreed that each one was much too stupid to be helpful. All three were simply bad guessers. With each one, after several meetings, the bad guesser would offer some particularly silly conjecture and I would thank them for their efforts, inform them that they weren't very good at their jobs, warn them that they were probably ruining lives, and then walk out their door.

Additionally, at my spouse's request, I met a half dozen times with a behavioral psychologist and with two highly-paid psychiatrists. I felt these people were skilled, but eventually neither they nor I could figure what, if anything, I needed to change. They were quite willing to take my money, but even they had to admit there simply wasn't much reason to. I really was and still am a decent fellow.

Still, I wanted to improve and I began using writing as a way to reveal what was hiding under my skin. Much to my surprise, I found a number of hidden things and soon symptoms were being explained by root causes. I started out slowly, but over time I began to develop some modest analytical skills and discovered the key to unlocking my

hy·po·der·mal

secrets was to figure out when I was lying to myself and why I was doing it. I had to move my ego to one side to let the truth appear.

While writing, I had some insights and shared them with my wife, explaining in the process of demeaning me, she was eroding her own credibility with our children. I tried to explain to her how important it is to not undermine a father's relationship with his children, even if the father was loaded with faults – ultimately it would come back to hurt her. It did.

I realized how important it is to children for parents to present a united front by delaying discussions of needed behavioral adjustments and solving disagreements in private. I suspected she couldn't know anywhere near to the degree I did that once a child loses confidence in a parent, the trust doesn't return without some serious effort and even then, sometimes it never does.

Nothing deterred my wife from her dedication in protecting our children from my perceived foibles. Dedication remains as one of her greatest strengths. Once she got something settled in her mind, it would take much more skill than I possessed to affect any change, but that didn't stop me from trying.

I wanted her to be beloved and trusted by our children, but over time, I realized that she was focused on the immediate need or demand of each child, unable to see the big picture in which sometimes allowing an immediate hurt was the right choice in order to avoid a greater problem later. She just couldn't understand that always reacting to every discomfort was making her feel better, but it was not teaching our children responsibility or consequences for their own poor choices. I begged her to stop because I knew this would come back to haunt both us and the child. It did.

The fact that my wife was missing this particular insight became crystal clear one day when my fifteen-year-old daughter was having a perfectly normal, but unusually

hy·po·der·mal

intense rage session. She and I had just enjoyed a shouting match and then gone to our respective corners to cool off. In the meantime, another problem had arisen between my wife and myself and I became focused on addressing and solving that. My still seething daughter overheard the discord and sought to insinuate herself into the discussion and hi-jack it in order to continue addressing her own frustration. This had become her modus operandi of late.

My mind was filled with clear, calm thoughts at that moment. I had long been aware that my daughter had not only been permitted, but even encouraged by her mother to exhibit disrespectful attitudes towards adults over the past year or so. She needed to be reasoned with and taught that she was being rude. I had made several attempts along the way, but it was hopeless as long as my wife was countermanding every effort.

My daughter was convinced that she had the right to commandeer a situation simply because she was filled with teenage angst. I had tried to help her see that was not a good thing on several occasions, but of course, being a perfectly normal teenager, she had raged on.

Attempting to continue my discussion with my wife was interrupted by, of all people, my wife. She accused me of abusing my daughter by not allowing her to fully express her concerns that instant. I explained that the worst thing we could do as parents would be to continue teaching our daughter that it is okay to behave as she was. I said that by acquiescing to her demands, we were de facto giving her license to behave like a brat. My entire family was witnessing this and what happened next stunned me into silence and stabbed me in the heart. The shock almost overwhelmed me.

My wife accused me of damaging all of my children by not allowing my daughter to freely express her anger whenever and however she chose. I tried to reason that she was a child and should not be given free reign until she had

hy·po·der·mal

better control. I was told I was wrong and then my wife declared for all to hear, that I was dangerous and abusive. She said I had scarred my daughter for life, quickly gathered all our children and told me that she was going to take them to safety, away from my damaging influence. Shoving the whole bunch out the door and into her van, I was left standing there with my mouth hanging wide open.

I am so grateful a family friend, an impartial witness, had been there and witnessed this entire fiasco. If not for him, I might not have been able to prevent darkness from crushing me, as it was, it was a close call. The man who had been standing to one side throughout the entire affair was a local priest and long-time friend to our entire family. I asked him what I had done wrong. To my surprise, he told me that I had done everything right and that he admired the way I had tried to calmly bring goodness into a very bad situation.

I had not raised my voice and never lost focus of calmly teaching my daughter and wife an important principle while simultaneously trying to solve a separate, touchy misunderstanding with my wife. I would have certainly assumed I had failed in some way, but for his honest assessment. While I grieved, he told me I had acted as well as he could have imagined anyone could have, much better than most, especially considering the pressure directed at me from two sources at once.

I could not believe that a mother would think that kind of communication would not harm her children and later said as much to my spouse. This was not well received and the relationship began to deteriorate at a much more rapid rate. My wife continued to insist that I was abusive and there was no rational way I could understand how she came to that conclusion.

I pressed for clarification, but not surprisingly there was nothing she could offer that didn't fit in with the normal give and take in a healthy family. However, my children being told they have to be taken away from their father because he

hy·po·der·mal

is a threat, when that is a lie, is highly abusive. I feared this kind of behavior from their mother would scar them and produce negative repercussions for years to come. It did.

I had many, many faults, but harming a child, in any fashion, verbally, emotionally, physically, or mentally was impossible and unthinkable to me. I could be angry and in the heat of a moment, but I could never intentionally hurt a child under any condition. Cruelty was never an attribute within me. I felt I was utterly innocent and genuinely betrayed.

I assume her motivations were good, but whatever her motivations, the reality was that my wife was destroying my relationships with my children. If I had to guess, I would say she was blinded by her frustration at me not meeting her own expectations.

Through the years I have learned that false modesty and arrogance are equally bad. I seek the truth about myself, whether positive or negative. The truth of the matter was I was a kind, good, and dedicated husband, but once I was certain that my wife was purposefully undermining my parental responsibilities, I began considering the most difficult choice of my life. I could see that our marriage was all but ruined.

Additionally, not only were my responsibilities being impaired, but the very fabric of all my family relationships were being destroyed. This realization was more than I could bear. I faced a hard decision. I could stay in the home to counteract the combined poison generated by my wife's undermining and the hypocritical actions between two married antagonists or I could leave and hope to affect good from outside the home. I decided to stay.

I have hated hypocrisy all my days and can't bear to have any hint of it in my own life, although I had to learn to live with a little of it in my professional life – I still hate it though. This attribute has made it necessary, although rarely easy, for me to admit my mistakes, both to myself and to

hy·po·der·mal

others in spite of embarrassment and consequences. With that in mind, I will now share with you possibly the saddest personal mistake of my life and by my definition, this one qualifies as a sin. What follows my sin will be an unintended mistake, but that didn't alter the consequences, it only mitigates my guilt.

The difference between a sin and a transgression, at least as far as I am concerned, is that with sin you know to do right and choose to do wrong. A transgression is doing wrong without sufficient understanding or time to understand why something is wrong. You know, the heat of the battle sort of thing.

When stressed and tired coming home from work, getting angry with the numbskull who cuts you off on the freeway is a transgression. Given a little time to think and under better circumstances you could ignore the idiot. Chasing the guy down, getting your tire iron out of your trunk, and modifying the fellow's fender is a sin. I think you can tell the difference.

Inevitable consequences follow both of these actions, but the depth of guilt and/or punishment can vary according to the balance required from justice and mercy. In other words, the more you want to hurt someone, the greater your own guilt. What I am about to describe, I had a moment of clarity to consider if my actions were the best I could do, realized I could do better, but chose to act poorly anyway. I define that as sin and although sin can be easily forgiven, forgiveness often has nothing to do with consequences. Here is the tragedy.

I was at a ballgame for my youngest son and was in the middle of light-hearted bantering back and forth with an umpire. The umpire decided he wanted to involve his co-worker and the two of them unexpectedly teamed up on me and things got a little vicious and quite personal. I didn't see that coming. Up until that point, I had no feeling of conflict, but had simply been responding with funny rejoinders just

hy·po·der·mal

as millions have done with umpires over the years. It is part of the game.

During one of our many exchanges, a mother of one of the boys playing, who had previously made it clear she didn't like me, stuck her two cents in to our exchange and castigated me, ordering me to stop harassing the umpires. She did not know that the umpires had instigated the negative tone she was witnessing. She was not one of my favorite people either and I told her to shut up and leave me alone. I confess that was not nice, but we had a history and I wanted to make it clear I didn't appreciate her butting in.

My youngest daughter, who was then seventeen, had just arrived at the game and witnessed the interchange between the woman and me. She didn't know of our history nor did she know that the two umpires had come to me with tag-team derisions a few minutes preceding her arrival.

I was not particularly upset with anyone at that time, but this daughter, the same one my wife had encouraged to insinuate herself rudely into adult situations, became increasingly upset with me. She began to tell me what I was doing wrong and that I was embarrassing her and myself.

My first response was calm and measured, telling her that it was none of her business and she didn't have all the facts. I then explained once again that it was not her place to get involved in correcting or interrupting adults. She never took correction well and now she was unstoppable.

She responded with increasing rudeness, certain of the righteousness of her position given what she had witnessed. I became increasingly irritated with her and soon our words escalated until she did something that she had done before and it was something I simply could not tolerate any longer. She threatened to call the police on me.

This is actually a very serious threat for adults in this day and age, but I didn't treat it that way to begin with. I have no excuse for my behavior as I immediately began giving her sarcastic grief by telling her that she should go

hy·po·der·mal

ahead and make the call. I offered to dial the phone for her and told her she would look completely silly involving the police in a simple disagreement. I confess this was infantile of me, although I have yet to find an adult that hasn't acted similarly at some time or another with a belligerent teen.

We were sitting side-by-side on a bleacher bench and she told me not to touch her. It was childish of me, but I shoved her two or three inches with my hip. Frankly, I was sick of her behavior towards me and the fact that she had threatened to call the police on me for trivial situations twice previously did not help. Of all the tempers in our family, this girl held the top spot, but I could be a close second sometimes.

What she couldn't know was that I was particularly sensitive to this threat. Our well-meaning schools had indoctrinated our children with their right to be protected from abuse. Of course this was a good thing until a child abused the right. Just a few years earlier, I had tried to stop a nasty boy from abusing some younger children at a park. The boy looked me squarely in the eye and said he would scream that I was sexually attacking him if I didn't leave him alone that instant. He was serious. I immediately left him alone and he continued abusing the little children.

On another occasion, my own fourteen-year-old son once threatened me with calling in the authorities, claiming abuse. I calmly and immediately sat down with him, carefully and sincerely explaining that if I was indeed guilty, he should report me and I would willingly take my punishment.

However, if he was merely irritated, he needed to know I would be arrested, jailed, and presumed guilty until and only if I could prove my innocence – all to serve his childish tantrum. I further explained that I would lose my job, we would lose our house, and very likely our family would be decimated. He was a smart boy, completely getting the

hy·po·der·mal

message and although we still had disagreements, he never used that particular threat again.

My daughter angrily left the park and I soon headed for home as well. Not long after I arrived, she came home. I decided I had to convince her of a couple of things. First, she needed to understand that threatening with the police, even if she didn't actually follow through, could result in someone overhearing and things could easily spiral out of control. And if she actually did it, I would be arrested and would likely lose my security clearance which would mean I would lose my job. I was the only source of income for our large family and felt very protective, even if the threat came from within the family. This obligated me to treat her threat seriously.

The second thing I felt was needed was that if she continued her belligerent and rude behavior, as she had over the past two years with me, I truly feared that my daughter would one day pick the wrong person to pull that behavior on and she would be badly hurt. A good father is not required to be a best friend, but a protector. I felt it was my job to prevent her from getting herself hurt.

As I walked toward her room I had a very singular sensation. This is important. I was still angry and I felt a strong impression that I needed to cool down before speaking with my daughter. I chose to ignore that wise impression and walked into her room with my demanding and angry attitude. That was my sin.

I very angrily told her she had to stop threatening me. She responded with typical teenage anger and yelled at me to get out of her room. I then stated that she had to stop treating adults the way she had been treating me and her older siblings. I warned her that someday she might pick on the wrong person and it could go very badly for her. As you can imagine, she did not take that advice very well because unfortunately, it had been delivered in anger instead of love. That was my transgression.

hy·po·der·mal

With the best of intentions, but with the worst of deliveries, I tried to show her what could happen if she angered someone who could simply overpower her. This was not planned, it just occurred to me as she was screaming at me. I grabbed her and held her tightly in my arms as she squirmed to get free. Of course I was much stronger and she could not free herself and began to scream for someone to call the police. This only strengthen my resolve to teach her that she needed to learn that she can't just rage without impunity.

I clamped my hand over her mouth. I knew if she continued treating people as she had treated me for the past several years, one day she would meet the wrong person and the consequences could be horrific, even deadly. My delivery method was terrible, but my intention was pure and I only meant to be helpful. Knowing what I know now, I would have simply hugged her, told her I loved her, and postponed the lesson for a better time. Another one of those might-have-beens.

Her brothers came running in and saw that I was holding their struggling sister. They reacted to what they thought was an attack. I sloughed off those good, brave boys and then took my hand away from my daughter's mouth. I had only meant to teach her that there could be severe consequences for treating the wrong person rudely.

As soon as she could speak, she shouted that I never listened and that I never just sat down to talk. I instantly let her go, erroneously thinking and genuinely thrilled she wanted to talk. She fled the room and ran to a friend's house, taking her brothers with her. Because of my own state of mind, thinking a bad argument had occurred and nothing more, I had no clue how far out of proportion this was going to blow.

From my sons' perspective, not understanding what I was trying to accomplish, our tussle must have looked and even felt like some sort of out-of-control assault. I was

hy·po·der·mal

angry, but I was always in complete control of my emotions and actions, using the bare minimum of force. I am told there was some bruising, but that was an unintended outcome from the struggle. I had never intentionally hurt any of my children, rarely even spanking any of them.

I mistakenly thought things had settled down, but I found out several months later my wife had contacted the police. She and my daughter had made an official report of abuse that day. My wife never spoke with me about the incident, assuming I was guilty of all that was claimed. This was revealed much later, when I was finally given the chance to explain the circumstances. I figured once the facts were made clear, all would be forgiven and we could work out our hurt feelings. Nope. Not even close.

Her response ranks as another one of those "worsts" I have endured. This one knocked me to my knees. She said she still considered me an abuser and would not have changed a thing regarding her involvement of the police. This was my greatest surprise and greatest disappointment in over thirty years of marriage. I knew that nothing serious had occurred. It had never been anything more than a strong disagreement, identical to what happened every day in thousands of families. I never dreamed that my wife would make such a devastating mistake in judgment. I felt like the proverbial rabbit shot with a cannon. Just fuzz and fur is all that was left.

I found out that I had been officially investigated and since there was insufficient evidence of child abuse, I was now in the public record "only" as a domestic abuser. My wife told me this news as though she had done me a favor. I had held my struggling daughter tightly and covered her mouth, something that had happened to each of our children in one way or another many times. That was the extent of my "crime." I do not deny I behaved badly, I just wish there had been more of a sense of proportion in this one.

hy·po·der·mal

    I loved and still love my daughter. An entire life and a spotless record of kindness and caring was blown to pieces and I was relegated to the legal title of abuser for holding my own misbehaving daughter tightly in order to save her from potential trouble. I believe she had been encouraged wrongly in this event. Once my wife told me that she thought I had been and would always be a potential abuser, I realized that all my triggers were now pulled and would never be unpulled regarding my marriage. I felt ruined.

    It nearly killed me (literally), but I decided the poisoning of my children as they witnessed the daily decay and rot of their parent's relationship was even greater than the damage my wife was inflicting by her actions. The hypocrisy was too much for my heart. In 2014, I left our home and moved into a small bedroom provided by that same priest who was a friend of the family, the one who had witnessed my wife "saving" her children from their "abusive" father who had given all he had to give to each of them.

    My own beloved father, confidant, and greatest supporter died just nine days later. Seldom have I felt more alone than at that moment. Only one of my children had shown any interest in my side of the event. The rest shunned me with some of them not coming to the funeral and others not coming anywhere near me. The misery of being away from all that was precious to me lasted for sixteen months.

    Now we come to the trough, the low point of my life, the darkest and most dangerous time I have ever lived. I never thought I would come close to feeling the despair I had felt as a seven-year-old abandoned by my mother, but this was close, very close. I suffered and wept day after day, feeling the life-sustaining presence and lives of my children drift away forever without my being there. I wanted to die and began to make serious plans.

    A short aside is in order before I unleash the totality of my misery. At this time, I was working for people who were

hy·po·der·mal

so confused that they demanded I only do things that were detrimental to our government. I became an expert at appearing to do work while avoiding any actual damage.

It was horrible and contrary to my morals, but I managed to keep going in each day. I was surrounded by people who had nothing better to do than hurt me professionally if they got the chance. Crippled by my broken back and scads of other maladies, my health was, for the first time in my life, lousy. I had lost my father and my family just days apart.

I was lonelier than I had ever been and this time it was coupled with the bitterness of missing my younger children as they grew up. The loneliness of "what might have been" is much more intense than anything I had previously experienced. I would come in from work, collapse in the same chair my father sat in for years, switch off the lights and turn on some quiet music, listening for several hours until I thought I could convince myself to sleep.

I had never in my entire life experienced trouble falling asleep. Previously, I could practically will myself to drift off within seconds of my head hitting the pillow. That changed. Every night was now a fight and I would spend between three and six hours lying in bed, wishing I was dead. Lack of sleep is deadly for the depressed.

After the weight of my darkness finally began to crush me, I started sitting with a loaded pistol beside my chair. I must have spent hundreds of hours debating how to die and what method would be best. Several times, I almost justified suicide by convincing myself my family would be better off without me. My children visited me only twice for a couple of hours during the sixteen months.

I could see that without me around to provide a detrimental target, maybe their mother would stop her destructive behavior. I considered thoughtful and clean ways to die as well as mysterious methods, often thinking it might be best to simply disappear. I dreamed of death and was desperate for relief.

I gave suicide the most intense consideration of my life, especially during the months when I had no hope at all. I thought about my death constantly and contemplated as many aspects of it as I could cram into my brain. Many years earlier, my father had died and returned. He shared with me his experience and although this is not the place to relate such an intimacy, suffice to say because of my faith in him, I have spent my entire life with no fear of death whatsoever. Death from suicide, at least as a practical matter, was not scary at all.

My hesitation came from the fact that I couldn't figure out a valid reason to kill myself. Every angle I examined was selfish and I concluded there was simply no legitimate, non-selfish reason to commit suicide. At least for me, there was one persistent thing that kept me from going over the edge. I didn't know for a fact that God loved me, but I believed it so strongly that I couldn't be shaken from my belief. It was just as though I knew, even though I didn't "know." I am not sure what to call this, maybe faith-plus?

I wasn't afraid of God's wrath or of disappointing Him. I had been a good father and believing God to be a father as well, I figured He loved His children much more than I could ever love my own. I knew I would only respond with kindness to one of my own who was suffering as I was and felt certain God would only do the same, except He would do it perfectly.

My hesitation was not from fear or guilt, but because I somehow felt God was so smart there simply had to be a reason for me to keep living, I just needed to find it. I allowed myself to think there could be something worthwhile I might possibly do in this world if I could avoid the coward's way out.

There were definitely times when I had no hope. The mental anguish could be overwhelming and it was during those hopeless moments that my belief in God made me wish for hope. I can't explain it, but apparently that is enough. God's love was not enough to save me because I knew he loved me even if I died. Simply wishing for hope when I had none was what saved me from suicide.

What I Just Tried to Say, but in Fewer Words

- You can only marry one thing at a time and still have any hope of your actual marriage growing and prospering. Sure you can marry your children, career, money, or many other things while remaining married to your spouse, but that marriage will, at best, remain stagnant.
- If you get a prompting, my advice is to heed it. If you don't heed it, the world doesn't come to an end, but you will have some highly preventable and nasty clean-up to perform.
- There is one tool left in the survival bag, even when hopelessness settles over you. Simply wishing for hope is enough and it will save your life. You don't have to believe this, just sincerely do it.

hy·po·der·mal

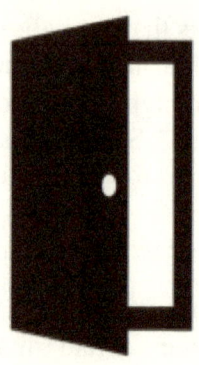

e·piph·a·ny

 You might think taking my finger off the trigger and walking away would be one of the greatest events in anyone's life, but not mine. Yes, it was a good thing, but what came afterwards was so incredible, that it dwarfed my brushes with death and made them look insignificant. I am going to share this very personal experience with the belief that you can either have a similar one or, failing that, piggyback off mine. Either way, you can't lose.
 After sixteen lonely months, I woke up one morning terribly depressed as usual and began pondering what I might be able to do with my solitary life to shake this depression. I realized that somehow I was going to have to find someone or something to serve. I stumbled through some scenarios, and finally the obvious hit me. Why don't I serve my own family?
 I packed up my few belongings and returned to my home with the determination that no matter what, no matter my personal discomfort, I was going to give everything I could for the welfare of my children. My reception was a little cooler than I would have hoped, but I didn't let that phase me.

hy·po·der·mal

My wife was iceberg cold and I realized I was going to have to give her lots of space. We had a big home containing several empty bedrooms and since I had just spent the last year or so living in a hundred square feet, I figured another bedroom would do me just fine. I settled in and determined to do some good.

The epiphany that is about to drop on me out of the blue is so important that I think I need to provide a little bit of point A to point B for clarity's sake. If nothing else, I hope to make it clear that most processes, including epiphanies, can be made very understandable with a little dedicated digging.

I suppose all that you have read up until this point is exactly that, a dedicated digging along the path that started with a four-year-old (point A) and now culminates some fifty-four years later (point B). Well, here goes my best effort to show you how an "instant" epiphany can be fifty years in the making.

In the summer of 1976, I started keeping a journal. At first it was more of a diary in which I simply recorded events, but it gradually morphed into a full-blown journal as I added feelings, insights, and lessons learned. I kept my journal faithfully and still continue to do so today.

I developed this habit from two influences: First, my father, because he kept a journal and gave me a blank one of my own when I left home and second, a wonderfully wise man named Spencer Kimball, who coincidentally resembled Yoda. Yoda is the green one. I had admired this man during my teens and he had promised me it would be a marvelous thing to keep a journal. I believed him, but didn't have a clue how marvelous it would prove to be or that it would play the life-saving role it did.

I hate to belabor my point A to point B efforts, so jumping to 2007, my job had become so dreadfully boring that I was struggling for anything to make the long hours pass. I was ensconced in a fishbowl of cubicles filled with co-workers who may or may not have had something worthwhile to do themselves. If I had to guess, I would say not.

To be completely truthful, we actually had tasks to do from time to time, just not very often and rarely of any value. Nevertheless, everybody was seriously devoted to appearing busy and I felt the same obligation. I needed something that mimicked work, but was actually interesting and also worth doing.

One day it came to me that I could transcribe forty years of journaling and the process would look very much like real work. I brought in one journal at a time and over the next year, I typed several hours each day.

You might stop and ask the question, "Why didn't you just ask for more work?" If you are asking, that is another excellent question. The answer is that in the environment in which I was employed, my management had very little to do themselves. To compound trouble, they had people foisted on them (like me) even though they didn't have any work to provide us.

At first, I peppered my boss with requests for work. I was constantly told "soon" or "in a while" or "it's coming." One day my boss seemed more than a little irked with me. It dawned on me for the first time that he had nothing to give me. I realized that I was only irritating him with my requests for work. I decided to stop and didn't speak to my boss, not even to say good morning, for three months.

One morning, as I was sitting with my feet up on my desk, reading the newspaper, my boss came to see me for the first time in many months. I was embarrassed by the compromising position in which he had caught me. True to my nature, I said, "Well, you sure timed that about as badly as you could." He smiled and said, "Oh, it is about to get worse. I am here to speak with you about your performance rating." Great. Just great.

hy·po·der·mal

This was my first official yearly performance appraisal. I had not done much of anything during the preceding twelve months. Don't get me wrong. I had done everything I had been asked to do to the best of my ability, it just hadn't amounted to much.

I was given a list of the things I was supposed to have done. I looked at them and cringed. Fortunately, I didn't say a word. My boss then started giving me a glowing report. He said that he hardly ever gives an "A" rating to a first year employee, but, and I quote, "your communication skills are so excellent that I feel compelled to award you the highest score." I had not spoken to the man in three months.

Now that I knew how the game was played, you can see why I never went into my boss's office to ask for assignments. He let me know that as long as I didn't bother him, I was in his good graces. Every now and then he threw a few hours work my way, but for years I was basically instructed to do nothing, be quiet, and take my paycheck.

This is not what I wanted to do with my life, but my family was large and we needed a large paycheck. While I was once wrestling with the morality of my job, my older brother shared an important thought. He told me that if I didn't occupy the position I did, somebody else would. He then said, "At least you are paying tithing and fast offerings, financing missions, and providing for a good family. You are not squandering any of the money on anything that is not worthwhile."

I thought about it and realized he was right. I determined then and there to do the best job I could, but to no longer worry about things I couldn't control in the work place. I wish I had figured that out about life in general, but that is coming.

I ended up working on my journals quite often at work over the years. My co-workers thought I was a superhero (I was always busy doing "something') and considered nominating me for employee of the year.

hy·po·der·mal

It was very rewarding and quite nostalgic reading over my life while noting my changes in perspective. It was also a little depressing in that I had recorded in excruciating detail quite an unbelievable number of steady failures.

At the completion of the transcription, I realized I had made a serious mistake. I had faithfully and perfectly copied each and every word verbatim, including misspellings and grammatical errors. I thought it would be fun for anyone reading my writings to see what a terrible speller I was and how poorly I had written. That was one really dumb thought. I decided I would go back through each volume and correct all my mistakes.

The corrections took a few months and once completed, I pondered the thought that as I had been faithfully transcribing, many details and insights had come to mind that I probably should have included to make the telling more interesting. I had not done this because I somehow got it in my mind that my actual writings at the time were sacrosanct and could only be recorded as originally written. This was another really dumb thought.

I decided to undertake a total rewrite, this time taking my time and adding every detail, thought, afterthought, observation, and conclusion that came to mind. I began transforming my words from a simple journal into a much richer life history.

Next, I realized that I had a ton of memories regarding my youth that were gradually fading with age. I had started my journal at age eighteen and that meant all of my early life would never be recorded unless I began right away. It took two years to gather every memory I could dredge up, including all that I could glean from family members. I compiled my findings and ended up with almost seven hundred pages of youthful stories and felt great sorrow that much had been lost under the dust of time. Oh, how I wished I had kept a journal as a young man.

hy·po·der·mal

After completing that addition, I decided to add photographs, important documents, maps, and letters to what was now a full-blown life history. I gathered pertinent stuff from everyone in my family and from my own keepsakes, scanned several thousand items, and pasted them electronically into the story.

At this point, I was dealing with seven volumes, a total of six for each decade I had lived, with a separate volume dedicated to my two years in Korea. The stories in Asia were rich and so numerous that they needed a stand-alone telling. The seven books were single-spaced and three to four hundred pages each. This had grown into a massive effort. My co-workers thought I was a superhero and considered nominating me for employee of the year.

I ended up re-writing every volume over ten times and possibly as many as twenty over the next few years. Truth be told, I am still not done. It has occurred to me I will likely pass away before I finish editing everything to my satisfaction.

One day while reviewing the writings dealing with the period in which I met the girl who became my wife, a funny little thought entered my head. I was now approaching sixty years of age and as I looked back on that innocent nineteen-year old boy, I cringed just a little bit. What on earth was a boy who was about to leave on a two-year mission, doing with a fifteen-year old girl? In retrospect, this appeared a little creepy.

As I sat and contemplated what was happening at that time, I was led back to my days as a high school senior and the girl with whom I had fallen in love. I re-read my thoughts and felt the same resentment that had haunted me during all the ensuing years. Why had she rejected me? What had been so wrong about me? Why wasn't I worth keeping? Why wasn't my best good enough? Why had she tried to kill herself? Was it my fault? I began to sink into an all too familiar funk.

hy·po·der·mal

I then had an experience like no other in my life. It felt as though an unseen force opened the top of my skull, dumped an entire and perfectly contained package of knowledge inside, and then slammed the lid shut. The thoughts came all at once and I realized for the first time in my life that I had spent my entire life making very deep commitments to people very quickly, much, much faster than other people. Girls, teachers, missionary companions, school chums, church leaders, and on and on, the pattern had been there all along and suddenly I could see it. This is important.

I clearly realized that time and again I had developed a much deeper commitment to someone than that same person had for me – and I had no clue that had been the case. I began to think about how lost I had felt when my first girlfriend had "abandoned" me for her life at college, leaving me alone. I had believed we would have continued forever. Now, I could see that she had done exactly what she should have. It was never abandonment. I was sixteen and she was eighteen and she needed to move into her new world just exactly as she had.

I then pondered what had happened to girlfriend number two, the first true love of my life. For forty years I had assumed she had not found me good enough and had cast me aside. I had envisioned our lives together, growing old. All at once I knew that she had not abandoned me or betrayed me at all. She had done exactly what a seventeen-year old girl should do – she had moved to the next phase of growing up.

Instantly, I understood something that had been entirely hidden from me for decades: I had literally spent my whole life making very deep, very rapid commitments and when others didn't manifest that same level of commitment, I felt betrayed.

Amazingly, the second that thought ran its course, wham! Another epiphany bowled me over and I saw that I

hy·po·der·mal

had an unusual approach to all relationships. Again, I never had a clue until that very moment my way of developing friendships was highly unusual and the vast majority of people took much more time to develop the level of commitment I so easily and quickly gave.

The old saying, "You don't know what you don't know" is perfectly descriptive of my life to that point. I didn't know that I was the one who was abnormal. I had spent a lifetime being confused that so many people, who I would have easily given a kidney to, didn't exhibit the same attachment and dedication to me. It dawned on me that throughout my life, as soon as it became clear that someone didn't have the same level of loyalty, trust, obligation, or dedication to me that I had for them, I felt betrayed.

These back-to-back epiphanies caused me to rethink my entire life. I spent the day mentally demolishing and reframing a lifetime of failures into successes. I didn't know it right away, but I was in the process of forever changing the way I would conduct my life from that day forward. We are talking a gigantic paradigm shift, but what most affected me was the incredible release from decades of guilt. The burden had been with me so long, I didn't realized just how heavy it had become and there aren't sufficient words to describe the relief.

The following day, the first thing I decided to do was to look over everything I had written regarding my missionary days because I suspected that all the misery I had experienced needed to be viewed with a different set of eyes. That was the one period in which I "knew" just about everyone had betrayed me to some degree. I began to examine the facts from the point of view that maybe I was the abnormal one. Holy smokes! An utterly different story unfolded right before my eyes. I was reading the words of a stranger.

I cannot describe how unnerving it was to be reading something I had written, read, and edited a dozen or more

hy·po·der·mal

times and suddenly, every word was unfamiliar. All these people in my past had only been doing what was normal and I was the one generating unmet and unreal expectations. I know "mind-blowing" is just an expression, but I came really close to the real thing.

The aspect that most amazed me was that I could clearly see how other missionaries had only been trying to help me out of my blindness. I was staggered by this revelation. Instead of serving with a bunch of selfish ignoramuses, I had worked with perfectly normal people who were doing their level best to deal with a misguided and confused young man. I had been the problem all along. This took my breath away.

With no hesitation at all, I threw out my entire seven volumes with their twenty-plus reviews and re-wrote everything, starting with day one. I probably had close to 300 hours invested solely in my missionary story and I chucked it without thinking twice. It was not the truth. It was not reality. At the time I wrote it, I believed every word, but my "truth" was based on a false foundation that I did not know was false and I would have defended it to the death as true, unshakeable as granite. I had built on sand.

I mention the rewrite of my missionary days because the EDS (Epiphany Derailment Syndrome) was not through with me yet. It was while my heart was filling with gratitude for all those young men who I thought had been my enemies, that epiphany number three hit and it was the tsunami of epiphanies.

This is the one that changed my life most profoundly. This was the truth that was so great that I cannot and will never be able to deny it. Because of it, I will never be able to commit suicide. Because of this truth, I will never be able to hate anyone and I will never be able to give up again. But let me make this perfectly clear, it removed none of the pain of living, it only makes it bearable.

It turns out that I had spent my life defining success such that there was no possible way it could have resulted in

hy·po·der·mal

anything but complete and total failure. The thought that unlocked this priceless understanding, revealed that the way in which I perfectly defined diamond-hard, unbreakable, genius-approved, and most importantly, God-sanctioned success was utterly and totally false. Until this truth was revealed to me, I could not have been convinced otherwise. There wouldn't have been sufficient language in the world to have swayed my certainty of a path that was killing me.

My problem was that I had a highly developed, lifelong, fully-embraced, flawless, all-encompassing, and untouchable understanding of success. With such an assurance, there could be no doubt in my mind that I was a complete and total failure. There was no room for debate, no room for discussion, and no possibility I was wrong. I knew this to be true because I knew exactly what success was and I wasn't it. I had studied success all my life and understood every aspect there was to know about it right up until I didn't.

I came to my unflinching certainty of being a perfect failure by having spent a lifetime studying the examples of others who had succeeded and not been failures. When it came to success, there was no aspect, not a single one, I had ever come close to achieving.

I read about heroes, great men and women who overcame tremendous odds, and people who had never faltered. I studied leaders and beloved individuals who were practically worshipped for their accomplishments. I knew and internalized what it took to be a great missionary, husband, father, grandfather, religious example, employee, driver, builder, and every other category worth trying for. I had catalogued, reviewed, and memorized numerous examples of all these successes and I never once came close to any of them. Not even in the same neighborhood.

My definition of success had been based on what someone else had accomplished. I figured that all I had to do was become what they had become and I too, would be a

hy·po·der·mal

success. This is an extremely logical approach. Monkey see, monkey do. The problem with this plan was that there was no possibility that I could ever become what they were. My plan was perfectly designed to fail in every way.

I mean a successful missionary was beloved by all other missionaries, wasn't he? I had seen this with my own eyes. He also learned the language flawlessly and quickly, served in all levels of leadership and was sought as the go-to fellow for advice and guidance. I achieved precisely none of these essentials for success and therefore, I had failed in every way possible. More guilt.

A religious example never makes major mistakes, even in private when no one is looking. He is filled with the direction at all times and because of his righteousness, he serves in capacities in which he affects hundreds, if not thousands of people. He never gets angry and always treats people with kindness. I failed in every way possible. More guilt.

A great professional knows tons about important things. He has accumulated a magnificent set of skills and is admired by all who work near him. He is even admired from a distance. He is in demand because he can do the job better than anyone else. He is trusted and sought after for advice. He is promoted to the top of any organization in which he works. I failed in every way possible. More guilt.

A successful husband is adored by his wife. He doles out advice that is perfectly valuable and solves problems without batting an eye. He never causes his wife discomfort and she can't wait for him to come home.

He is always kind and tender, never losing his temper and keeps his worries and problems to himself. He is a paragon of virtue and the exemplar spouse for every other wife that knows him. I had seen these men myself and I achieved exactly zero of these essentials to merit the title "Successful Husband." I failed in every way possible. Guess what? More guilt.

hy·po·der·mal

Ah, now, a successful father! That was my only real goal in life. Money, accolades, awards, and luxuries, none of these things mattered by comparison. Sure I had wanted success in the mission field, also as a husband, as an employee, and a myriad of other things, but fatherhood was the only thing that really counted for me.

A successful father is constantly sought by his children for sage advice and important guidance through the pitfalls and alligator-filled swamps of life. His word is equivalent to scripture and every bit as inspiring. He is funny, loved unceasingly, and never, ever forgotten.

He only speaks with wisdom and is the first person his progeny wanted to see when arriving home. He never speaks in anger and is perfectly in control of every situation. Basically, he can do no wrong.

I had witnessed fathers performing at this level and try as I might, I never came within a mile of hitting a single one of these essential characteristics. As you can imagine, being a dismal failure in every way imaginable as a father, I was a perfect candidate for suicide since this was really the only thing that mattered to me. The guilt was almost more than I could bear. In fact, sometimes it actually was too much and I believe God must have sustained me.

My third epiphany blew away all my false truths. Now, I understood that all I could do was the best I could do given the skills that I possessed while living under the conditions of a given moment. Give me another set of variables, I might do better or I might do worse, but I could only accomplish whatever my best effort at the moment would allow.

It was actually crazy to have defined success in the way I had. There was no other outcome possible but complete failure in trying to achieve the same things another had achieved without possessing the same tools and circumstances. It was impossible. I finally understood what it meant when I heard true success was in the trying, not in the doing.

hy·po·der·mal

We are solely responsible for performing our given role in a process to the best of our abilities given what we understand at the time and rarely, if ever, control outcomes. Don't misunderstand, we absolutely influence outcomes, but we do not control the outcome itself. Even our responsibility for outcomes is limited as long as we sincerely tried to do well. My job had been to be the best boyfriend or missionary or husband or father I could be under the circumstances of that time. You know what? I had done just that.

I mistakenly thought I was responsible for each and every one of my unfavorable outcomes, even though I never had any control. My responsibility was only to do the best I could in the process, but when it came to the result, I demanded the credit, it belonged to me and me alone. Much more lethally, I owned the guilt of each failed outcome and it belonged to only me as well. This misunderstanding nearly killed me. I had wasted years smothering under the weight of a million supposed failed outcomes, none of which I had any possibility to control.

If you don't think the previous two paragraphs were very meaningful, you might consider rereading them. They may be the most important in this book. When you think about it, almost all of the grief in your life comes from believing you had some control over a result in which you never did.

What I Just Tried to Say, but in Fewer Words

- It was the desire to serve someone or something that set me on the right path. It didn't fix a thing, but it made all the difference.
- You may not have the same unrecognized characteristic I did, abnormal commitments, but that doesn't mean you don't have some characteristics to expose and understand. Want to know what makes you tick? Follow the pain.

hy·po·der·mal

- Unreal expectations are at the foundation of most of your misery. Ease up. Rethink. Forgive yourself for most, if not all, of your supposed failures – particularly if you really weren't trying to fail. They weren't failures at all, it was just you doing the best you could under the circumstances. And that is the very definition of success.
- What I didn't know was that I had logically and rationally picked the worst thing I could pick to establish as my definition of success: Someone else's success. That had seemed so smart at the time.
- Our responsibility as mortals is to do the best we can, given our current tool set and the situation in which we are plowing through. Our input will influence the outcome, but we have zero control over the outcome itself. For goodness sakes, stop grieving as though you did.

P.S. Just so you can know how dumb I can be, I want to let you in on a secret. Sixteen years before I had my epiphanies, that same law student who had made such an impression on me in college, had told me the main cause of my unhappy life. He said that I made friends very fast and very deeply, but then reacted badly when others didn't respond to me in the same fashion. He pointed out I had unreal expectations of others. I believed every word he said and promptly ignored them because I didn't recognize their importance. At least I never forgot them. You don't have to be dumb for sixteen years if you choose not to be.

hy·po·der·mal

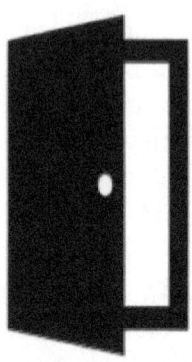

fail·ure

Six decades of unquestionable and proven failures instantly evaporated. What would I do if I was no longer a failure? First of all, I had to rethink every facet of my past, present, and future. In the process, considering my particular set of attributes, I started to recognize my own successes far beyond what I could have ever believed.

Once I clearly understood the challenges I had overcome and the way in which I had responded to those challenges, for the first time in my life, I could sincerely pat myself on the back. This was something I had never done before and had avoided even considering. What perfect failure ever congratulates himself?

With a new understanding of my world, I was ready to try to solve every problem in the known universe. I began approaching events from the new perspective that I couldn't control the outcome and I could only control my own role in the process. I completely stopped worrying. Wow! Did that ever free up some time in my daily schedule! I renewed my efforts regarding my marriage, thinking that if I was the problem, then I would do everything within my power to change that.

hy·po·der·mal

One afternoon, after several hours of fruitless conversational recycling and miscommunication, my wife stated, "I can only accept part of you and the rest is unacceptable." This was followed by (and I repeated it back to her six times to make sure we were communicating accurately), "I am afraid to give you what you ask for because I think you will use it to justify staying the way you are and not improve." Stunning! Her opinion of my current status, my integrity, and my desire to improve was much lower than I could have guessed.

I tried dozens of times to explain that being accepted for what I am today doesn't mean I won't improve tomorrow – in fact being accepted, respected, or appreciated for the person I am today will certainly motivate me to be a better husband and father. I must have stated ten times, "I need to be loved and appreciated for who I am today, not just for who I can be someday."

With my new understanding, it was very easy to avoid anger during this discussion, but my wife became increasingly frustrated and soon grew abusive. I begged her to stop and leave me in peace. She wouldn't and increased her intensity and volume, so I left the room. On my way out, I heard her murmur and complain under her breath about how once again I had taken a positive thing and turned it into a negative. When I'd heard her say this before it had dumbfounded me. Now I realized she was simply unable or unwilling to see things from any point of view but her own. This insight filled me with sorrow.

I felt a glimmer of hope a few months later, when something happened that I had given up on ever coming to light. My wife admitted she had purposely undermined my relationship with my children over the past years. I was surprised she did this because I had long been asking for her to acknowledge her role in the failing relationships and she had steadfastly denied any role in the least.

hy·po·der·mal

I immediately forgave her and was quite willing to put this behind us. She said she would try to do all within her power to make things right again and repair the damage she had done. Sadly, she may have very well done her best, but nothing got better and the bad things continued. But this time, I knew I had no control over the outcomes and simply continued to do the best I knew to do. As things crumbled, I felt peace in the midst of my sorrow.

I shared with her the deep and sensitive truth that my only real goal in this life was to be a great father. I said I also wanted to be accomplished at other things such as being a great husband, but my greatest desire since I was a young boy was to be a beloved father. I confessed to her I thought I had failed, but then I realized I had done the very best I could and how my children felt (outcomes) was out of my control.

I described how when I first became aware that she was consciously tearing at the respect and position I had with my children, I took that very hard because that feeling is so tightly linked to the thing most important to me. Her betrayal had added to my conviction that I had not lived up to any of my "success" goals. I then stated I no longer felt depressed.

After her confession, I explained that I was fully aware that I had not been the greatest father in comparison to other great fathers, but I had done about the best I could, given my own set of skills, problems, circumstances, and so forth. I then revealed to her that this point was really the root of all our disagreements. I felt good about my efforts, but all her communications indicated I was falling short.

I'd spent years struggling to convince her to "stop trying to change me." This had been my way of saying I am doing the best I can and if that is not good enough, we are in trouble because I can do no better under current circumstances.

The failure of her expectations would have been difficult enough to deal with all by itself, but as I learned that she had knowingly transferred her feelings into my children, my despair had increased until it became unbearable and that had been the reason I had left our home for sixteen months. I had come to believe I would never meet my wife's expectations because she seemed to only want me if I could be something other than what I could be.

Now that I understood my failures weren't failures, they were actually successes and my definition of success was actually certain and unstoppable failure, I continued doing the best I could, but this time I wasn't concerned with outcomes or results. EVER. I realized that I had no control over my wife's responses and therefore no matter what happened, I didn't feel inclined to take credit for the bad or the good. Of course, that was only true if I had done the best I could under the circumstances – which sometimes is not very good at all and that's okay.

My life became increasingly peaceful and I discovered a condition that was far more important than being happy. I learned that I could be at peace while completely surrounded with chaos and bedlam and no longer had to react to every negative thing that happened in my life.

Of course, just because I was at peace between my ears, that didn't mean that my life was not crumbling down around me. It just meant I was no longer depressed and had some ability to rise above my sadness and focus on what good I could accomplish or at least attempt to accomplish in the midst of trying times. I was no longer wasting time worrying about "what ifs" and could now put all my energy into bettering the "what is."

Things in my marriage went on exactly the same, no improvements for two years, in spite of my new wisdom. I lived in my own bedroom with my relationships not anything like I had hoped they would be and yet I continued to function at a fairly positive level. I wasn't happy, but surprisingly it wasn't nearly as important to be so. I left the outcomes in God's hands.

hy·po·der·mal

Without my new truths, I am certain I would have returned to the darkness and spent my time trying to reason out a good death for the perfect failure of my life. Instead, I just kept plodding along although nothing regarding work, my health, or my family relationships really improved. In fact, just about everything grew a little worse. Somehow I kept a good attitude, seeking good wherever it could be found while letting the bad roll off, unabsorbed.

There were still serious mistakes being made by my wife as she seemed unable to stop tearing at my connections with my children. I believe she thought she was doing right, but much like me with my incredibly wrong definitions of success, she was acting on a rotten foundation and didn't know it.

I tried many, many times to speak to her using a variety of approaches, but all to no avail. Because I knew I wasn't responsible for the outcome and it was actually easier to keep doing the best I knew how. I trusted God would take care of the results and I was fine (meaning at peace, not happy) no matter what they were. I didn't and still don't hate her for doing what she believed to be right, but I didn't and still don't trust her either.

It is critical to allow someone to accept a truth only when they are able to be responsible for knowing it. A four-year-old may know how to start a car (truth) but that doesn't mean he should be given the car keys. Knowing the truth before you are able to wield the power of the truth can be devastating to the knower and to innocent bystanders. I had to let my wife continue her behavior, even though I held the keys to fixing our marriage.

One night, something so horrific occurred that I knew a change was required. I was reaching out to my same outspoken daughter, who was then twenty-one years old. She brought up the event in which I held her down five years earlier. I referred to it as a wrestling match and she spun up with anger, thinking I would never understand her point of view. I knew she had very, very deep and dark feelings towards me, but up until that moment, I had no clue just how dark.

Even though she was an adult, I never felt she was fully responsible for her anger and hard feelings. If her mother had not encouraged her in her rudeness and then supported her interpretation of our conflict as abuse with the necessity to involve the police, I am certain we could have readily overcome our difficulties just as millions of other families had under similar circumstances. Sure it would have taken work, but without the support of my wife and with her corresponding misguided influences, it was never going to be possible.

That daughter had always been my favorite in a sense because of her strong personality and the need for my protection. Even as a toddler, she had consistently rubbed her brothers and sisters the wrong way. They often ganged up on her and expressed their anger for her arrogant and abrasive nature. I heard complaints about her almost from the day she was born and had spent her entire life defending and shielding her. Often literally. I only loved her more and more because of this.

It wasn't that I supported her bad behavior, I just understood that she was strong-willed and needed an intelligent touch to guide her into productive and likeable paths. In that respect, I had been anything but a failure. I had done everything within my power to keep her safe and happy, but I couldn't control the outcomes. During all her pre-teen years, she had been my buddy and we probably spent more time together than all her siblings combined.

It broke my heart when my buddy rejected me over our one argument and I had become deeply depressed over that "failure," using it as one of my main reasons to consider suicide. I mean how could I have failed her when she needed me most? This time, now that I understood the real definitions of failure and success, I hoped I was equipped to

hy·po·der·mal

deal with almost any situation. I was, but I still couldn't control the outcome.

The horrific thing that night was that my daughter completely lost control and screamed at me to die, to go to hell, and to [pick your profanity] myself. The more she screamed the more out of control she became. She told me that she had been advised by law enforcement that at any point she could report me to the authorities and I would be immediately picked-up and punished. She said she desperately wanted me to go to jail.

Several family members were present during this meltdown. The one thing I can feel good about was that I was in complete control of my feelings and actions. I responded calmly to each attack, only seeking to make some aspect of her life better.

The poor girl dug into the past, revealing she had blown our previous conflict into something huge and monstrous. She claimed I had hit her, pulled her hair, and blocked her from leaving, none of which had happened. She appealed to her brothers to support her as witnesses, but they told her none of what she was claiming had happened either and that she was remembering things that simply weren't true. She grew more and more angry. Her mother didn't help one bit and even tried to support some of the false claims, particularly the hair pulling. Any hair pulling was completely inadvertently done.

During her abusive tirade, I pointed out to my wife that this behavior is the result of her supporting our daughter's misbehavior over the years. I went on to say that now she was witnessing the very horror I had been trying to prevent, a young adult with no manners, respect, or control when angry.

My daughter refused to discuss anything in a civil manner and shouted that she would say anything she wanted whenever she wanted. This was not her fault as far as I was concerned, her mother had done things to transform my

hy·po·der·mal

beautiful, but headstrong daughter into someone who could be a danger to herself and to others. Sadly, my wife's chickens had come home to roost and my beloved daughter, my wife, and I would all pay the price.

I realized that I had to make a decision once again. My daughter was fully capable of fulfilling her threat to have me arrested, whether I was guilty or not would not matter to her and maybe not to the legal system. I had been reported once before by her and documented as a domestic abuser and this made any report a credible threat. I couldn't afford to lose my ability to provide for my family.

Additionally, I still dearly loved my screaming, out-of-control daughter and I didn't want her to do something she would regret for the rest of her life. I also didn't want her to be uncomfortable and I realized I needed to leave our home again so that she would have a place in which to feel safe.

My marriage had been dead for some time at this point. The only reason to stay was that I had three boys still at home who I loved more than life itself. I wondered what might be the lesser harm in this situation, leaving my boys with all the associated pain that would cause me or staying and thereby forcing my daughter to suffer with the possibility of me getting thrown in jail.

I was first and foremost a protector and so I made my choice and moved out. Again. My boys didn't seem broken up at all about my decision, but I can assure you I was giving my pain-wracked, abandoned seven-year-old a run for his money. I left, never to return. I was at peace, but I wept for days.

When I was big into misdefining success, I made lots and lots of lists. Here is a list of my life's failures to date, all of which will miraculously become a list of my life's successes, think of it as a two-for-one:

1. I grew up without a mother.
2. My mother didn't want me and abandoned me twice.

hy·po·der·mal

3. I was abused by my aunt and uncle.
4. Women didn't like me as a boy.
5. Girls didn't like me at all during my youth.
6. I spent much of my youth isolated.
7. My step-mother hated me and got me kicked out of my own home, forever.
8. Girlfriends rejected me.
9. I was a terrible missionary.
10. The only girl who would marry me wanted another fellow.
11. My wife accused me of being a religious hypocrite.
12. My entire professional career has been based on nothing and is littered with bosses and co-workers who hate me.
13. My business failed.
14. My health failed.
15. I suffered from depression for five decades.
16. My wife undermined my relationships with my children.
17. I have a chronic broken back.
18. I was falsely reported to the police as a domestic abuser by my own wife and daughter.
19. My wife didn't want me unless I was somebody else.
20. My marriage failed.
21. I left home for sixteen months and nobody missed me.
22. I desperately wanted to commit suicide for years.
23. I returned home after sixteen months and nobody cared.
24. Many of my children don't have much to do with me.
25. I failed as a father.
26. My daughter despises and hates me.
27. One of my sons hates me and one despises me.
28. I left home to never return and nobody minded in the least.
29. I have never served in a trusted capacity in my church or my community.
30. I live alone in a single bedroom of someone else's house.

hy·po·der·mal

31. I have no home and very little money.
32. I seldom have visitors and basically no one seeks my company except when obligated.
33. Rarely does anyone in my family contact me.
34. My current job is a nightmare and my management hates me.
35. I tried to reconnect with my mother in my fifties and she rejected me a third time.
36. I am horribly lonely as I write these words.

You might wonder if I believe it when I say the above is really my list of successes or if I am just blowing smoke. It is my genuine list. Nothing changed on the outside, but something really important changed on the inside to make this the identical list of both my successes and failures. However, IT IS NOT my list of happiness. Success and happiness are no longer connected in my mind.

Yes, growing up without a mother was difficult and although I had suffered much, it ultimately was the key to my contentment. Your path may include a mother and if that is the case, I hope she plays a wonderful role in your own search for peace. I could not have made the journey I did without the start I was given. Each rejection in the list all felt real and some actually were, but none of them had to determine how I would treat others or how I felt about myself. Failure? No way.

My career really has been about as awful as it could be short of being a con man, but I have always provided for my family, regardless of my personal suffering. I met all of their needs and even most of their wants. Failure? No way.

Just because people didn't meet my expectations doesn't mean I have to hate them or love them any less. Sure, we have to have expectations of people. We would be crazy not to, but we don't have to let their performance affect how we feel about them. I have learned to be at peace and to love independently of my own or everyone else's failures and successes. This is really a great way to live. Failure? No way.

I used to believe that lots of "stuff" was necessary for my happiness. I no longer believe this and as I have let go of the stuff of my life, I find that I much more easily sustain and live in peace. I miss my family terribly, but I understand I can't control how they feel or act with regard to me. I cannot emphasize enough how my sadness has not changed and yet completely changed when viewed through peace. It's like it can no longer affect me and I am free to devote all my heart to making things improve rather than lamenting the past and dreading the future. Failure? No way.

What I Just Tried to Say, but in Fewer Words

- Being at peace in no way makes any of your circumstances any better or worse, it only makes them bearable. The upside is that it allows you to use your limited abilities to focus on making things better rather than wasting time on what might have been.
- During any process, if you are giving about the best you've got to give considering all things, you simply cannot call the outcome a failure. However, all bets are off if you don't try.
- There are days that just breathing is the best you can do and that is a heck of a success. I know, been there, done that.
- No, I am not lying or deceiving myself or you when I say with a straight face "my failures are BY FAR my greatest successes." I only thought they were failures, they never were.

hy·po·der·mal

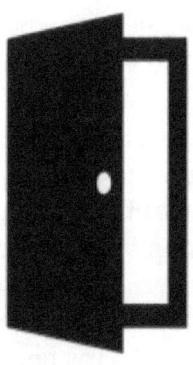

suc·cess

As of this writing, I find myself once more lonely and isolated, re-instated in the little bedroom of my friend's house. No family. Lousy health. Terrible job. This time I am experiencing a loneliness of a different kind. This time I understand that I actually have done just about the best I can and every outcome has always been out of my control. I don't mean to imply I didn't make mistakes, but the vast majority of the time I made good choices and when I didn't, I have tried to make up for my mistakes, doing everything within my power to set things right.

Of course, I am sad with most of my outcomes, but I am not what I would call depressed. It turns out you can be a total "failure" and still be content. Likewise, someone can be truly successful as all get out and still be miserable. My greatest sorrow no longer consists of guilt or worrying over disappointing results. My greatest sorrow now comes from not doing my best (given…) to prevent as many "might have beens" as possible.

I already lost sixteen months of my children's lives and that had pushed me to the very brink of suicide. Now I am missing most of my two son's remaining youthful days and all of one daughter's. No day can ever be recaptured, but if you are not there, they can't even be recalled. I have wept during the long nights and still tear up often. However, even when filled with sorrow, I am strangely at peace. The truth revealed by my epiphanies is so powerful that I am unable to backslide even though I am still willing to try. And very foolishly, often do. The truths, now that they are sunk deeply into my soul, are simply unstoppable, in spite of my weaknesses.

After my headstrong daughter left for school, I briefly considered moving back into my home, but in speaking with my wife about the idea, something very undesirable manifest. She told me she was happier without me around and this was not the first time she had said this. When I had returned after my sixteen month hiatus, she confessed that she felt safer and more secure without me in the house. I knew I had never been a threat and would never be a threat, so I had discounted what she said. This second time, I paid attention to her desires and did not return.

I continue to treat my wife with generosity and kindness, but I am also careful to not let her hurt herself by hurting me. I still feel an obligation and desire to provide and protect her and all my family. Some of my relationships with my children have deteriorated, but I know I have done the best I can and completely understand I can't control what results from my efforts.

As of this writing, I am at peace although nothing, not a single significant thing, is the way I would like it to be. I am not happy, but I am content. I would like many, many things to be different, but if nothing changes that is still okay. I hardly recognized the man in the mirror anymore.

Now we have come to the end of our journey. Apparently, I had failed at everything I had ever attempted and still I was a complete success. It has taken a lifetime of constant sadness and some close calls, but after all of these experiences, it has been worth it. I have finally learned to appreciate the here and now, regardless of the outcomes.

hy·po·der·mal

It is crystal clear that all my failures saved my life and then further rewarded me by showing me how to feel peace in every second of every day. I am one of the most skeptical people I know and I would have belittled you into tears if you had told me this was possible just a couple of years ago.

For me to learn to live without guilt and depression, all I had to accomplish was four things and these same four things will work for you, although you will have to tailor them to your own circumstances:

1. I had to stop linking my expectations to my love – especially love of self. I have maintained my expectations for both myself and for others, but I can't love any less when they are not met and yes, this is important too, I can't love any more when they are exceeded.
2. I had to recognize all of my faulty and completely impossible expectations and stop them. Although not as important as unhitching your love, getting rid of these boondoggles will keep you from a world of unnecessary hurt and unnecessary guilt. Guaranteed.
3. I had to recognize that every success I counted on was based on faulty definitions. If you are filled with guilt and circumstantial depression, you most likely have some rotten definitions for success (or failure). If you have any comparisons in your definitions, they are toxic. No exceptions. You only have to do the best YOU can do in a given set of circumstances with what you have to work with. Sometimes your best is just so-so. I promise you, heaven celebrates over so-so. Probably more times than not.
4. I had to understand that I had allowed every bit of my happiness to depend on outcomes I could not control and each success had been unachievable. I was absolutely doomed from the start. No wonder I wanted to die and felt constantly depressed. You do not control

the outcome except when you try to fail. Duh, don't try to fail. Success really is in the trying.

I no longer want to die. I still find living very, very difficult, but every minute is precious to me (granted, kidney stones make some minutes a little less precious). My career, my home, my family, my friends, my health, and every aspect of my life continues to be nothing like I want them to be and I am fine with that. Now, I do all I can to make things better, but am no longer concerned about results in the least and in the process I have found that which is most precious, peace.

What I Just Tried to Say, but in Fewer Words

- Success has nothing to do with outcomes.
- My life has not turned out in anyway how I had hoped it would be. In fact, it is utterly miserable and yet, I am completely at peace.
- I hope you can see just how poorly I have understood life as I lived it.
- My pain is very hard to bear, but it is no longer overwhelming and it never can be again…even if I want it to be.

hy·po·der·mal

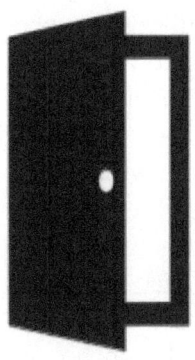

hope·ful

There actually are a few things that can guarantee successes or failures, depending on what you are in the mood for. Oddly, I find myself enjoying my failures more than my successes now. I know, I know, you are rolling your eyes just as I would have not long ago, but I promise you it is true. I have come to understand that failures are actually essential and at least in my case, the failures are proving to be much, much more interesting than my successes. But remember, this is only the case when I am giving a fair effort in the process. Shoot for failure and you will rarely be disappointed.

The difference in my feelings comes from viewing my outcomes through an attitude of peace. It no longer matters to me if I am happy, I would much rather be at peace. Shortly before I wrote this book, one of my sons committed suicide. Amazing doctors managed to restart his heart after an overdose and he is still with us, although it is really a day-to-day experience. A few months later, another one of my daughters became confused and told us she wanted to die and disappeared for a little while. She did not go through with her thoughts, but we had a real scare there.

hy·po·der·mal

In the midst of both of those experiences, I felt at peace. I spent my time trying to make any aspect of these events better. I comforted others and spoke words of hope because I was comforted and felt hope rather than despair. I understood the outcomes were not in my control and I could focus on what was possible before me because of the peace in my mind. Let me tell you, this is pretty powerful stuff and it is a great thing to face tragedy with courage and love unfeigned.

As you now know, I spent some years courting the Grim Reaper myself and even my brave father told me that things once got so bad for him that he decided to die, but was interrupted by a very inexplicable intervention. He said that just as he was pulling the trigger, he heard a voice clearly say, "I love you." He was standing alone on a solitary knoll in a Nebraska field. He never claimed he knew who spoke, just that he heard the words clearly.

By the way, the night when I finally ran out of juice and was deciding to live or die, my phone rang and that too, was a very inexplicable intervention. A man I had just met once was on the line and said he had felt impressed to call me. These things may not always happen, but I am convinced there are often powers at play we simply don't understand. There may be such a thing as coincidence, but it seems all too often to occur in a pattern.

I guess what I am trying to say is that depression and thoughts of suicide seem to be a common experience for many of us as we struggle through our weaknesses and yet each and every one of us, assuming we have our faculties, possess the tools to overcome these dark desires.

If I have done a good job, you now have some idea about how to go about finding the value in yourself regardless of the fact you have failed in every way conceivable. Sometimes it is the false definition that gets you. Sometimes it is in the attached expectation and your love diminishes when it simply didn't have to. Especially the love and respect for yourself.

Often, it is hate that drives us to our doom. A person who hates themselves is forced into one of two courses when faced with someone who loves them.

- Course One: They have to convince themselves that all the people who love them are crazy – which is what I did. After all, they kept telling me I was a success. How stupid. Didn't they realize what a perfect failure I was? This allowed me to continue hating myself and providing permission to sabotage all my relationships.

- Course Two: They have to admit they themselves are the crazy one for hating themselves because everybody else loves them and everybody is right. I finally found out I was crazy – or at least the definitions I lived by were crazy. People really were right to love me. I was worth loving. I no longer hate anyone, not even myself.

Sometimes it is simple confusion that gets us. You have now read the story of my failures and hopefully can see how I became so confused. I felt a compelling need to commit suicide and struggled with depression all along the way. I know your life hardly resembles my own, but our experiences have much in common and it is my greatest hope that I have told my story well enough that you or someone you love can relate and rise out of the ashes just as I have.

My greatest hero once said, "Father, forgive them, for they know not what they do." I appreciated that thought and even imagined that I understood the concept, but I couldn't begin to understand how to apply such an unbelievable ability into my own life. I was simply too busy hurting and hating on my own cross to love those hurting me. Once I discovered how to be at peace in the midst of pain, I found that not only could I understand, but I even began developing

hy·po·der·mal

just the slightest ability to forgive others and (gasp!) myself. This has been a hoot and gets easier with practice.

I still suffer with my broken back and what I am about to say sounds like snake oil, but it isn't. After seven long, miserable years, I had the chance to have my spine repaired. I thought about it a long time and finally chose not to do so, largely because living with this difficulty has changed me so profoundly that I want to see how far it can take me. I truly love the pain now, although I really, really don't like it, if that makes any sense. There is no doubt that it continues to school me and helps me to be a better and more peaceful person. Well worth the price of admission.

What I Just Tried to Say, but in Fewer Words

That was a short chapter. Nevertheless, please consider re-reading the Course One and Course Two paragraphs again if you can. Pay particular attention to the comment about sabotage. This will explain some previously inexplicable behavior in people you know who are suffering. They are forced to sabotage or to admit they are crazy, so many lash out at those who love them. Knowledge is power. Use it!

hy·po·der·mal

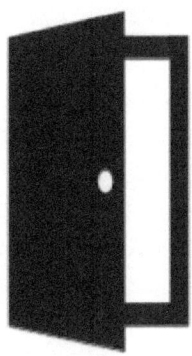

five·true·things

    I am glad you didn't skip to the end, because without having gone through all we shared, I am pretty sure these five things wouldn't have the slightest chance of becoming profound truths, the kind that once you know, you simply can't backslide from. Here they are:

1. Don't allow the love of yourself, a stranger, or anyone else vary with your expectations. Falling short is the very definition of being human. Throw in a faulty expectation or two and you've got a real mess on your hands. All hate stems from failed or faulty expectations with emotions attached, especially hate of yourself. I promise this is true. Here is the cool thing. If you unhitch this just a little bit, you will immediately see a benefit. I repeat, immediately. This is not one of those "feel good" ideas in which you have to guess if it works or not. It always works. Every. Single. Time.

2. If you or someone you know is considering Lie Driven Suicide, it is for one of two reasons or possibly both. Either they are viewing life as a snapshot or they have outcomes linked to their faulty definitions for success and failure. Regarding snapshots: When all hope fades

hy·po·der·mal

it is because you are no longer seeing your life as dynamic and it has become a still-shot that you sincerely, but falsely, believe will always continue stuck the way it appears at a given moment. Usually a really lousy one. Snapshots are a lie. Everything changes, sometimes for good and sometimes for bad, but as I have hopefully shown you, even when everything in your life falls apart, you can still be at peace. Life is an analog video and never, ever, a digital snapshot. Never. If you think things will remain the same, you are wrong. The outside may appear unchanged, but as your inside changes, everything changes. It's okay, I didn't believe this either until it happened.

3. Never tangle up outcomes with your definitions of success and failure. Success has nothing to do with an outcome. The only definition of success that counts is in doing the best you can, given what you've got, in a particular circumstance. If you had told me that it would have taken a perfect record of failure all my livelong days to succeed, I would have treated you like you believed in crop circle logic. I knew, ABSOLUTELY KNEW, I was a failure all my life. There was not the least smidgeon of a doubt because, my outcomes all screamed failure. When I discovered that some of my most spectacular failures were actually superhuman successes, I stripped every gear in my brain trying to process the thought. Please don't forget, if you shoot for failure, you will probably never be disappointed.

4. Peace, not happiness, is the cure. For you mathematicians: Peace plus sadness minus happiness still equals peace. In other words, peace is independent and supreme.

5. When you run out of hope, wish for hope. It will be enough. There are forces at work that more often than

hy·po·der·mal

not will provide you with just about anything but what you think you need. This is particularly true regarding happiness. In spite of this being a completely bizarre and illogical phenomenon, you will receive exactly what you actually need, exactly when you need it. Belief is not required and doesn't seem to particularly help anyway.

hy·po·der·mal

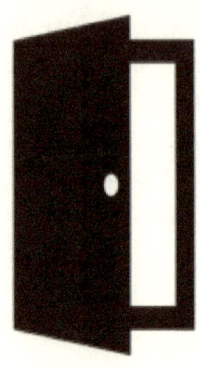

short·cut

    I may be wrong, but I am pretty sure there are no shortcuts when it comes to circumstantial depression and suicidal thoughts. That doesn't mean changes can't be made rapidly, but you still have to go through a process of discovery.
    I showed you that I had been given bits and pieces along the way that could have fixed some of my troubles, but it wasn't until I sloughed my way through all the steps that I was finally prepared to give away all my favorite stupidities. Many of us clutch our worst behaviors like boat anchors as we flounder in a sea of despair. I sure did. Getting rid of these obviously unnecessary things is the closest thing I know to a shortcut.
    It is my hope that as you read through the process of my lifetime battle with depression and suicidal thoughts, you will unlock the necessary insights to finally and forever get rid of these two diseases in your own life and in the lives of those you love. It is within your power.
    I assure you, there is no chance that I am anybody special with some peculiar set of skills. This should be obvious to you as you just read how I stumbled blindly along, leading face-first directly into boxing ring filled with

hy·po·der·mal

pain and misery. And yet I did it. If an average person like me can do it, you can too.

Besides my own experience, I can give you one thing I did not have. I didn't understand how the root causes and my feelings of suicide and depression were connected. I hope this helps.

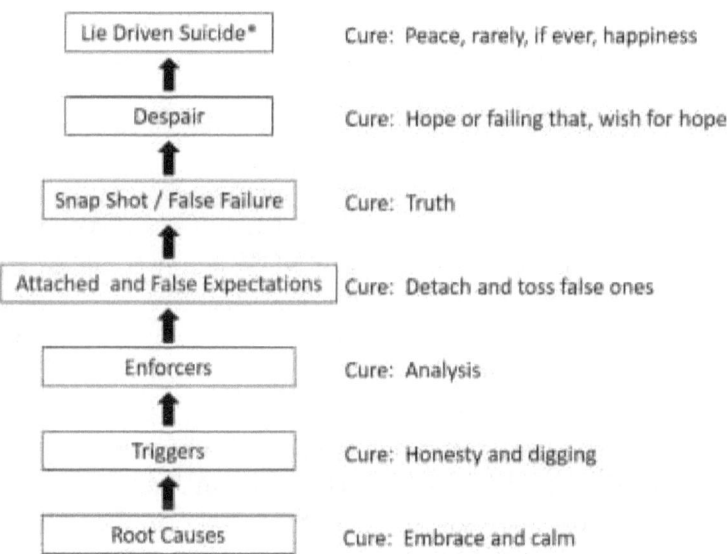

*Also works for Attention Driven Suicide and Circumstantial Depression

hy·po·der·mal

dis·til·la·tion

Lie Driven Suicide and Circumstantial Depression have two causes, snap shot thinking and false failures. If you ever expose these lies to sunlight and KNOW the two causes are lies, you will never commit suicide, just like you would never willingly chop off your own arm. You know that act is stupid, based on lies, unnecessary, and incredibly permanent. No upside.

The amazing thing is that you will also become content, BUT NOT NECESSARILY HAPPY, in fact, you will probably have plenty of things to be sad about. We all do. However, now our sadness fits right where it is supposed to be, not overwhelming us. Peace, not happiness, is the key to living inside your own skin. If it helps any, I didn't believe a word of any of this until I did. I am going on my fourth year of peace now.

The truth is that most of the time I am sad and don't have a whole lot to live for, but on the other hand, I no longer have anything at all to die for. It turns out that having lots to live for is not nearly as important as I thought it was and it is enough to be alive and to try to make some aspect of my own life or anyone else's a little better. The trying is the success.

hy·po·der·mal

I have no idea if this book will make any difference in your life, but that is an outcome and as we've discussed, I have no control over outcomes. My success is in revealing truths in the best way I know how to present them, not in what happens afterwards.

Hopefully, these truths will be part of the input in your own process. Don't be concerned about your outcomes, the success is in doing the best you can with what you've got at the time you are trying. Please, please don't link your well-being to things you can't control (i.e., just about everything).

Something like "good luck" might seem fitting as a closing comment, but that is really not appropriate at all. This stuff really works. You don't need luck, good or bad, you just need to work through the process. I guess I'll just leave you with

                    Good Life,

                                  Dark

hy·po·der·mal

You just read the gutsy, gritty version of my life. If you want to fill in the gaps with laughter, take a look at my book

Light Years by Dark Myer

This book is pure fun, but still has deep meaning scattered throughout the pages. If you look closely, you'll spot the tears between the chuckles.

www.ingramcontent.com/pod-product-compliance
Lightning Source LLC
Chambersburg PA
CBHW031418210526
45464CB00005B/1950